The Palm-Aire Spa

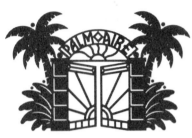 *7-Day Plan to*

Change Your Life

The Rejuvenation Program—
Diet, Fitness, Relaxation & Beauty

Eleanor Berman

Prentice Hall Press • New York

Published by Prentice Hall Press
A Division of Simon & Schuster, Inc.
Gulf + Western Building
One Gulf + Western Plaza
New York, NY 10023

PRENTICE HALL PRESS is a trademark of Simon & Schuster, Inc.

Library of Congress Cataloging-in-Publication Data

Berman, Eleanor, 1934–
    The Palm-Aire spa 7-day plan.

    Includes index.
    1. Reducing diets—Recipes. 2. Reducing
exercises. 3. Beauty, Personal. I. Title.
II. Title: Palm-Aire seven-day plan.
RM222.2.B456 1987   646.7′042   86-25263
ISBN 0-13-648361-5

Designed by Lucy Sisman

Manufactured in the United States of America

10 9 8 7 6 5 4   3 2 1

First Edition

Acknowledgments

This book would not have been possible without the help of many people. My sincere appreciation goes to all the people at Palm-Aire who make the Spa so special—and who contributed their enthusiasm and talents to the book.

Special thanks are due to Carol Upper, director of the ladies' spa, who was supportive from the start and did so much to help make the book possible. Thanks also go to Bill Freeman, director of the men's spa, Ken Kasten, vice-president, the World of Palm-Aire, and Lorraine Abelow, public relations representative, who were all so cooperative throughout the project.

Most of all I want to acknowledge the staff specialists whose expertise is reflected here. First and foremost is Fitness Supervisor Pam Schutte. Without her, there simply would be no book. Others who have shared their knowledge so generously include Tim Patton, Palm-Aire's talented nutritionist, whose wizardry turns low-calorie menus into treats, and his assistant, Karen Manno, who helped put the recipes into writing. Peggy Fisler, Sanford Bates, Marla Kaufman, Charles Breher, Carolyn Voce, Sylvia Ritchie, and Karen Consiglio are others who contributed their special know-how, as did all the members of the Palm-Aire fitness staff and Kay Clifton, who guided the illustrations for the exercises.

Finally, thanks are due to my agent, Connie Clausen, and my editor, Gareth Esersky, who made the idea become a reality, and to Creative Director J. C. Suarès and photographer Elizabeth Watt (with Karen Hatt) who transformed my bare typewritten pages into a handsome book.

Contents

Foreword

This is a book about renewal—renewal of mind and spirit as well as body.

Diet and exercise, though certainly important to us at the Palm-Aire Spa, are only part of the benefit of spending a week here. Feeling better—and feeling better about yourself—is our ultimate aim for you, and that is also what we hope you will accomplish by reading this book.

When the Spa opened in 1971, we were one of the first in America to pioneer the idea of a new kind of spa vacation for men as well as women. In these stressful times, those who come to the Spa are often as much in need of relaxation as weight loss. They are busy people who have found it hard to fit an exercise regimen into their lives, however good their intentions. They are people whose life-styles frequently call for eating out or eating on the run, making it difficult for them to stay on a prescribed diet.

They come to the Spa to "shape up" in every way, to leave their various stresses behind, and to concentrate on their personal needs for a while. Our goal is to demonstrate how good it feels to change your way of living, how energizing it is to get your body moving, and how easy it is to lose weight while eating nutritious, satisfying, low-calorie meals. We teach not only physical exercises but techniques to help control stress when you return home, and we try to inspire some serious thinking about how to feel and look as good *all* the time as you do at the end of a week at Palm-Aire.

These are the techniques, developed by our talented staff, that we will share in the pages ahead.

We are proud of the long list of prominent people who have visited—and revisited—us over these years, people such as Elizabeth Taylor, Liza Minnelli, Mary Tyler Moore, Goldie Hawn, Phyllis George, Coretta Scott King, Pat Kennedy Lawford, Mr. and Mrs. David Rockefeller, Paul Newman and Joann Woodward, decorator Carlton Varney, designer Pauline Trigère, and golf pro Nancy Lopez. When people who can afford to go anywhere choose your spa, you know you are doing something right.

But we are equally proud of the lesser-known thousands who have visited and left handsomer, happier, and healthier for their experience.

We hope you will find this book a head start toward this same kind of renewal.

KEN KASTEN
Vice-President, The World of Palm-Aire

The Palm-Aire Spa
7-Day Plan to Change Your Life

Getting Started

If you have been on—and off—dozens of diets, this book is for you.

If you're always talking about exercising—but don't *do* any exercising—this book is for you.

If you are feeling tired, depressed, and overstressed, if you don't like the image that looks back at you from the mirror each day, this is a book that can change your life.

For more than fifteen years, the Spa at Palm-Aire has attracted prominent guests, including some of Hollywood's brightest stars, for a week-long program of rejuvenation from head to toe.

Many guests have asked for the Spa's secrets. Now, for the first time, you can share them in the exclusive 7-Day Spa Plan outlined in this book, a plan specially adapted to be easily followed in your own home.

With guidance from Palm-Aire's experts, you will be thrilled to see how much you can accomplish on your own in 1 week. Along with the fabulous Spa menus and exercises, you will learn Palm-Aire's special techniques to help you relax, pamper yourself, revitalize your appearance, and refresh your outlook. You'll even learn how to make your surroundings feel special, just as they do at the Spa. All it takes on your part is the resolve to set aside time to follow the Plan carefully for just 7 days. To make it easier, each day's activities can be divided into short segments that will fit into your normal schedule.

You'll find that the Spa Plan is different from ordinary diet-and-exercise plans you may have tried. There are many good reasons why so many people are choosing to spend their precious vacation time at a spa—and why it is worth your precious free time to follow a spa plan at home.

The first is simply that spas respond to human nature. They know nobody will stick to any diet or exercise program without some strong motivation. The pampering for which spas are noted—the wonderful massages and facials and relaxing water therapies—serves a serious purpose. Because it makes you feel and look better, and eases the aches and pains of unaccustomed exercise, the pampering means you are more likely to stick to your new good habits long enough to see concrete results.

Your 7-Day Plan includes delicious personal beauty treatments, instructions for home facials, and even some massage strokes that you can do on your own, as well as suggestions for relaxing water therapy right in your own bathtub. These are the desserts you earn by sticking to the "main course" of the regimen.

Since it is not human nature to want to stay on a restricted diet on your own for very long, the Spa meal plan is designed to teach you how to eat *well* and still lose weight. Your menu for this week will consist of three delicious multicourse meals a day, an "eat rich/stay thin" nutritious low-calorie diet that will not only take off pounds now but lead to sustained weight loss in the weeks ahead. It will prove to you that you *can* eat satisfying meals and still lose weight by changing the kinds of foods you choose and the way you cook. Unlike most diets, this is a way of eating you can live with forever.

But diet without exercise will not accomplish what most of us wish for when we think of losing weight. Even if you take off a few pounds, the flab that widens your waistline and hugs your hips will disappear for good only if you melt it away with exercise. At home or away, beginning exercise means stiff and sore muscles. But like spa-goers, you will be motivated to keep at it when you see inches as well as pounds begin to disappear within a week, the result of a changed diet coupled with the proper kind of exercise.

A well-rounded program includes several types of exercise. Aerobics are most important. These oxygen-burning exercises use the body's large muscles. They not only strengthen your heart but also quicken your metabolism—the rate at which your body uses calories all day and even while you sleep—thus speeding up weight loss. And they help pare down those hard-to-budge fatty deposits on the body. The only way to metabolize that fat is to convert it into the energy needed to move your muscles, and aerobic exercise is the most efficient way to do so.

Other kinds of exercises also play a role in making you look better. Calisthenics and strength-building exercises help tone and shape the body. And stretching exercises are vital to ease tension, keep your body limber, and prevent injuries.

You'll sample each type during this week of intensive exercise, which has been designed to get you started on habits that can become a regular part of your routine. What's more, you'll learn that exercise can help you *feel* better within one week. Our bodies were intended to move—in fact, they break down from *lack* of use. In a matter of days your own body will begin to respond as it begins to move regularly. Put in one concentrated week literally to get you over the sore spots in a hurry, and in a very short time you can experience the wonderful exhilaration that comes with getting your body going. It's the kind of high that will motivate you to *keep* going when the week is over.

What else is special about a spa program? At Palm-Aire, where thousands have come to discuss the problems of staying in shape, we have learned how much mind and body go together, how much learning to like yourself more can help you gain control over your life as well as your weight. Following guidance from the Palm-Aire staff in the pages ahead, you will do some serious thinking this week about the barriers and mental blocks that are preventing you from becoming the person you want to be, and you will consider some of the options that might make your life more rewarding. Time for yourself, time to soak in the bathtub or relax during a facial, can be the time you need to take stock.

The treatments themselves will reinforce your resolve, giving you a little daily lift every time you look into the mirror and see your improved appearance—just the kind of morale booster that motivates you to do even more about changing yourself.

Stress can be another major roadblock to good intentions. It may divert us from doing the things we should to take care of ourselves properly. Activity itself is a stress reducer, something a week-long spa regimen will prove to you. The Spa regime also teaches ways to cope with stressful situations, common-sense techniques you can practice at home to help you relax and stay in control instead of letting stress take over.

As you follow the Spa's four-part Plan of menu control, proper exercise, relaxation techniques/beauty treatments, and time to examine your life and how to improve it, you will realize why the Spa Plan can do more than simply help you lose weight. It can help you to feel better overall than you have for months, or maybe years. All the parts of the Palm-Aire Plan work together as a whole to provide a sense of true renewal and inspiration to change your life-style permanently.

A good spa aims to be a motivation center reinforcing good intentions, generating new attitudes and behaviors that will continue to enrich your life long after your week on a spa plan is over. One important way this is accomplished is through education. Spa guests learn, often for the first time, exactly how the body functions—how it reacts to stress, inactivity, different types of exercise, and different types of foods. This know-how comes from talks by staff specialists—experts in nutrition, diet, exercise, beauty care, and stress control—whose knowledge is shared with you in this book. Rather than setting out a rote plan, each chapter that follows will help you understand how and why each part of the Plan works. You will learn how you can help your body do its job more easily and effectively—and make yourself feel and look better at the same time.

Recognizing how difficult it can be to find both the time and determination to stay with a fitness regimen amid the distractions and temptations of everyday life, Spa guests are helped to formulate a concrete personal plan at the end of their stay, one that can continue to work for them at home. You will do the same at the end of your 7-Day Spa Plan, determining ways to continue your good start as part of your normal routine.

A healthier, happier life-style can begin for you with the Palm-Aire 7-Day Spa Plan—but this will happen only with commitment on your part. Those who come to a spa have invested a week of their time and energy, as well as money. In order to reap the full benefit from a home spa plan, you must also invest time and energy. You may schedule the activities and treatments according to the demands of your own days, but for this one week, the Plan must take priority in your free time.

Of course, it's nice to be able to get away to a spa, but you can't always get away when you need it most. And no matter how marvelous your spa vacation, you still must come home and fit your new habits into your old environment.

The Palm-Aire 7-Day Plan is an introduction to the benefits of a spa without leaving home. It is also an answer for the many who have been to Palm-Aire and asked us for a refresher course at home. It can be a head start toward a greater sense of well-being and a slimmer body—your chance to invest one week in yourself and reap lifetime dividends.

4

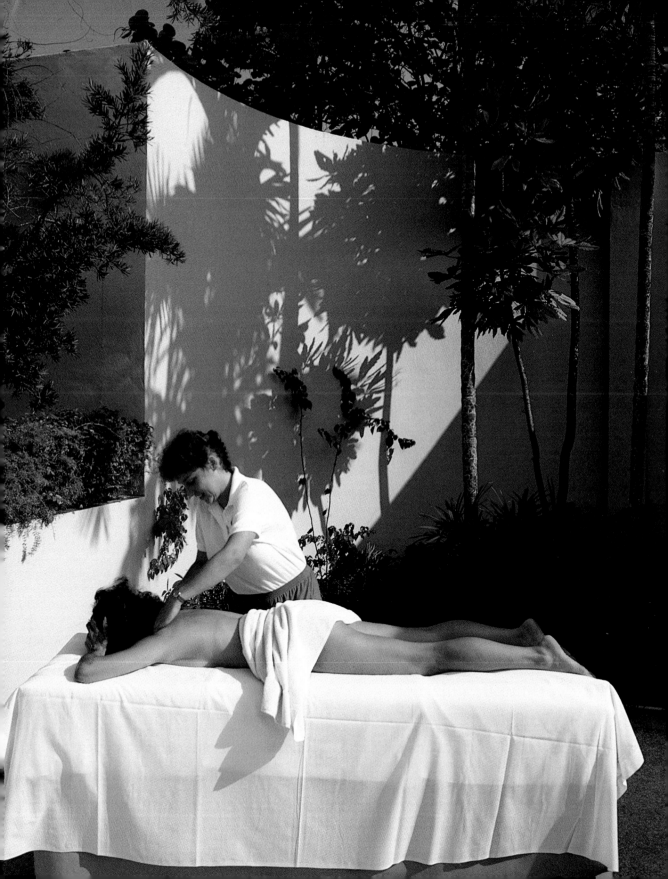

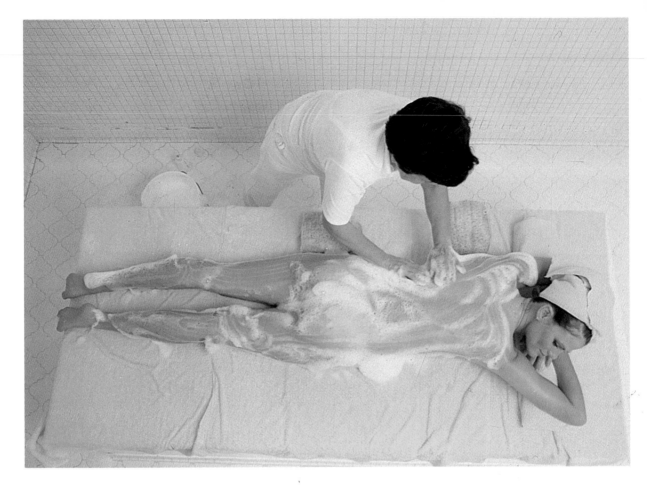

PREVIOUS PAGE
A soothing massage in the balmy Florida breeze
(Photograph by Elizabeth Watt)

ABOVE
An avocado oil and salt loofah rub gives an overall,
exhilarating glow. *(Photograph courtesy of The World of
Palm-Aire, Inc.)*

RIGHT
Soothing herbal wrap *(Photograph courtesy of The
World of Palm-Aire, Inc.)*

OPPOSITE
Whirlpools soak away worldly cares. *(Photograph
courtesy of The World of Palm-Aire, Inc.)*

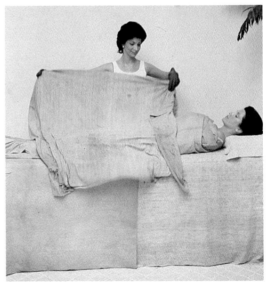

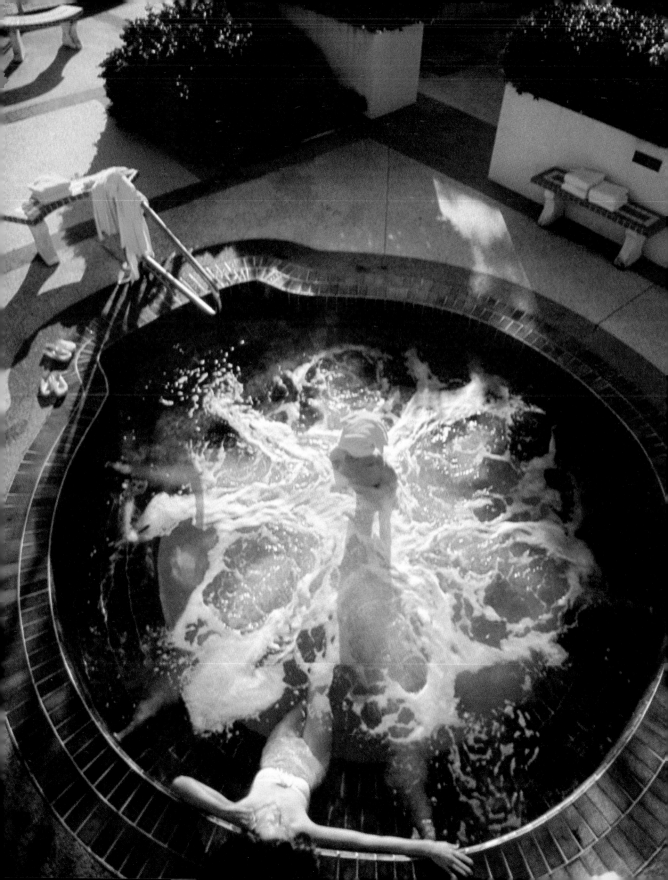

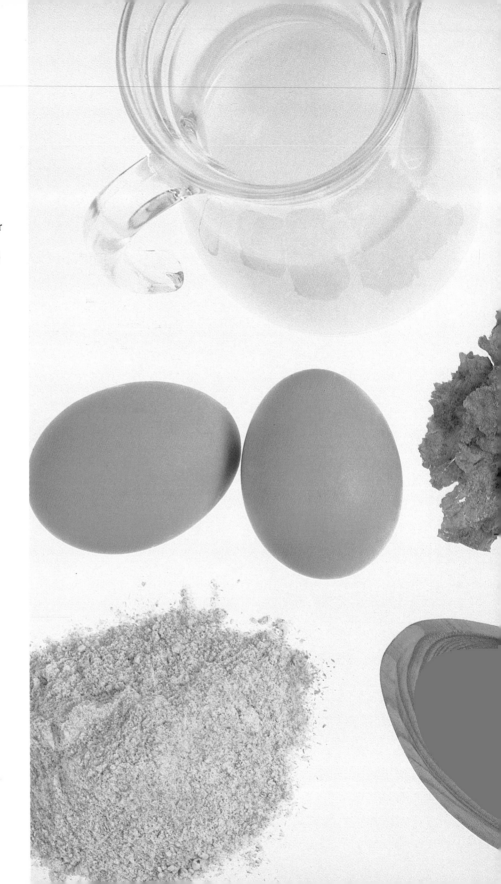

Healthful ingredients for
delicious Bran Muffins
*(Photograph by Elizabeth
Watt)*

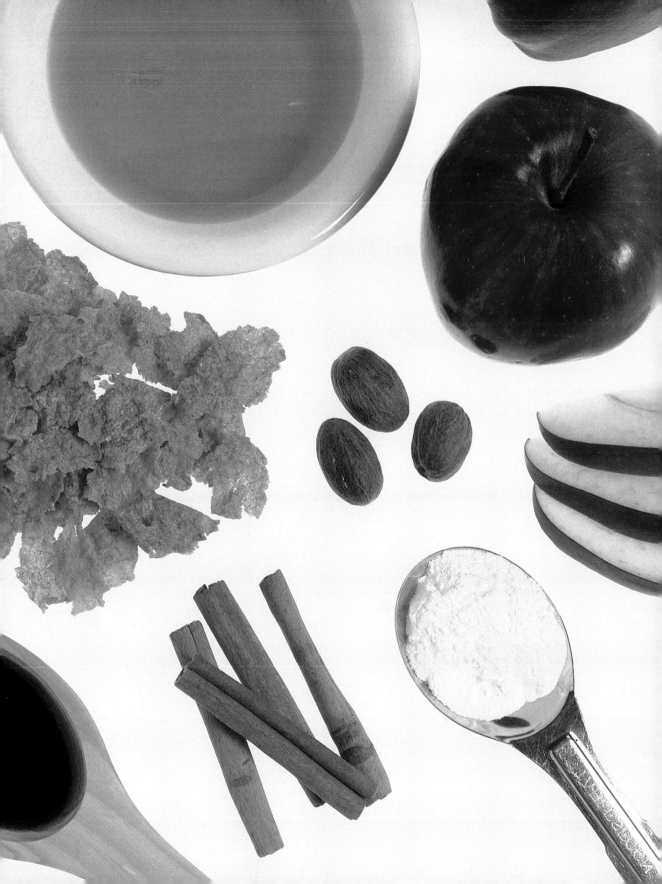

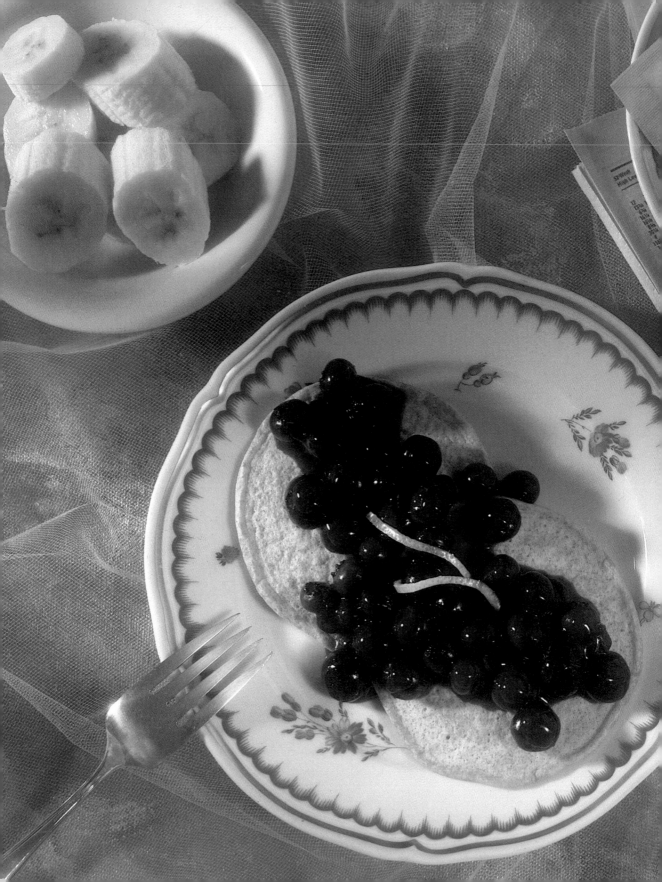

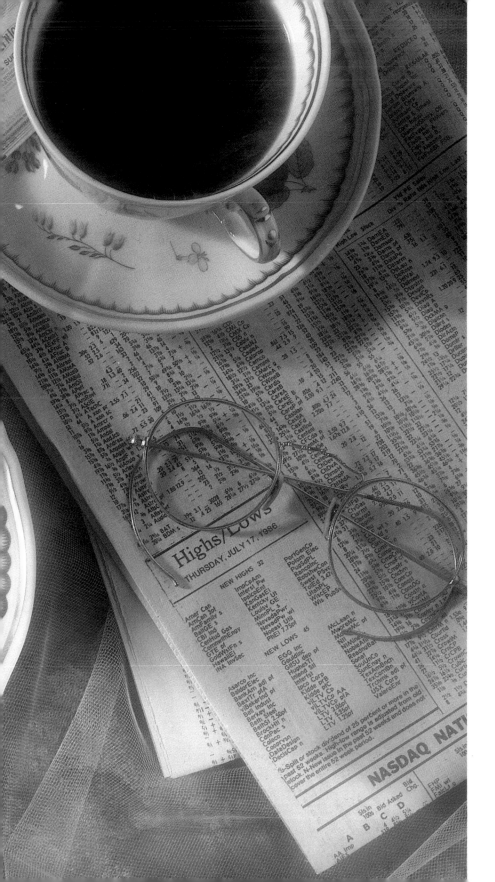

Breakfast menu: Buckwheat Pancakes with Blueberries • Sliced Banana • Decaffeinated Coffee *(Photograph by Elizabeth Watt)*

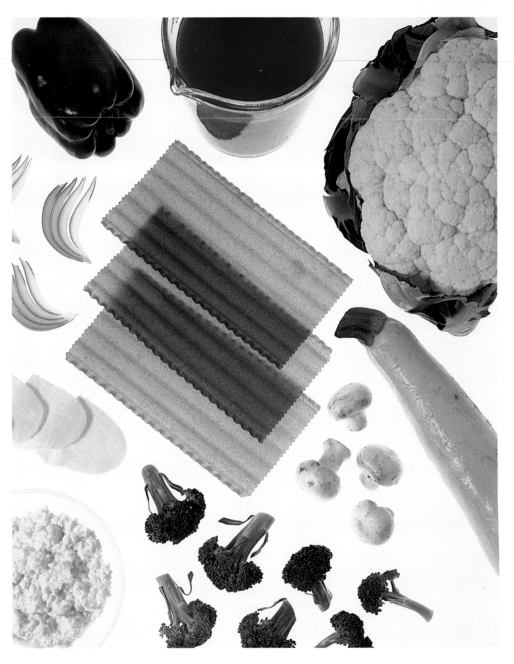

Garden fresh ingredients for Vegetable Lasagna *(Photograph by Elizabeth Watt)*

Lunch menu: Leek Soup • Stuffed Zucchini with Fiber Dressing • Tomato and
Onion Salad • Lemon Sponge *(Photograph by Elizabeth Watt)*

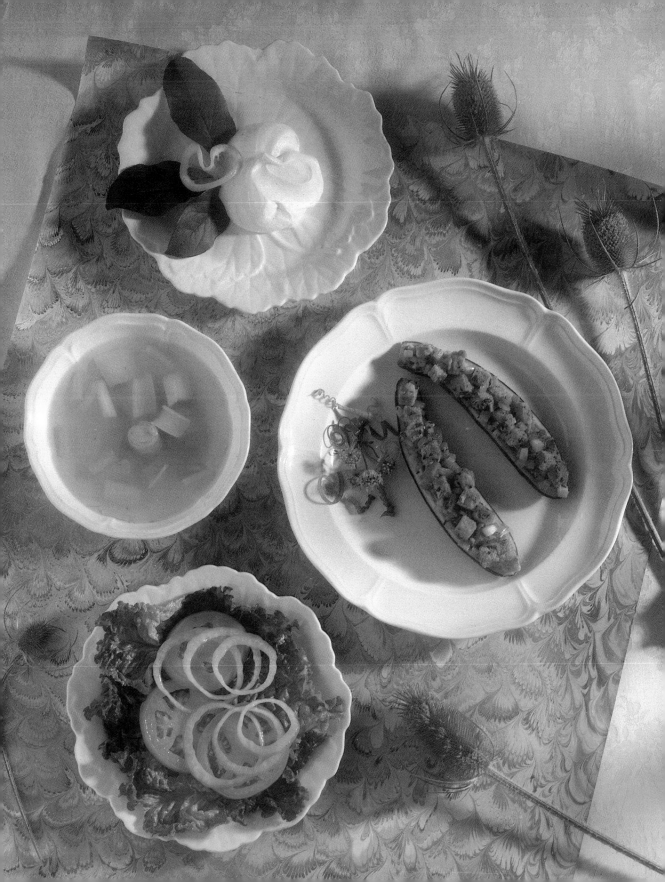

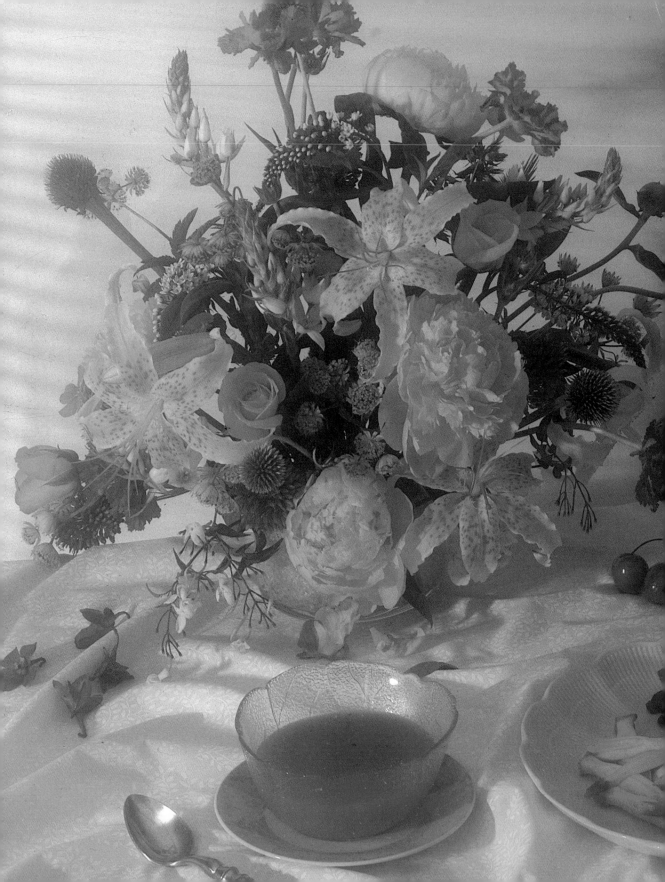

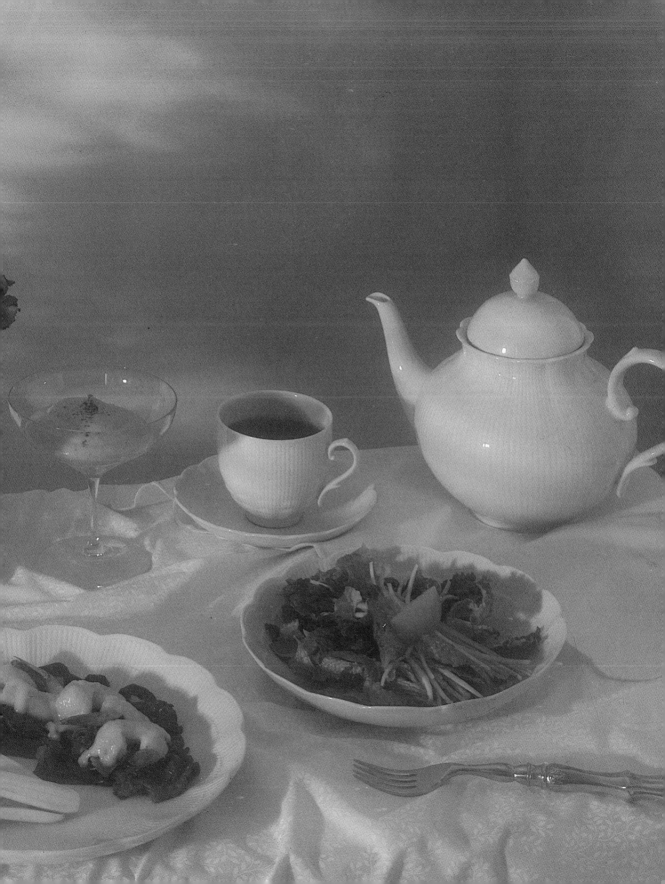

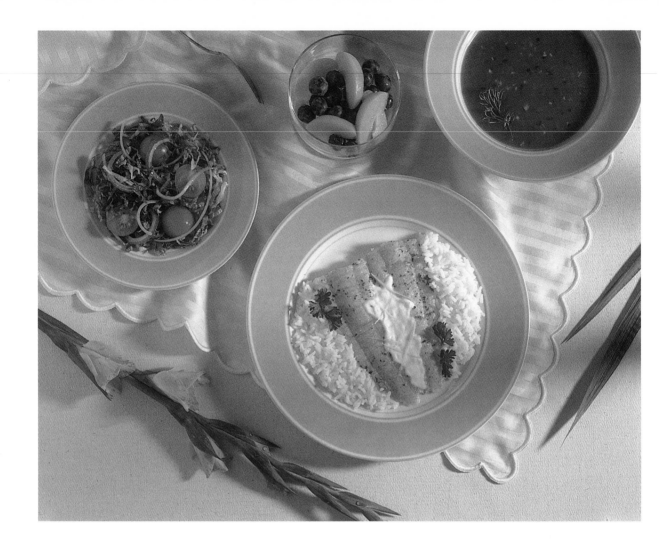

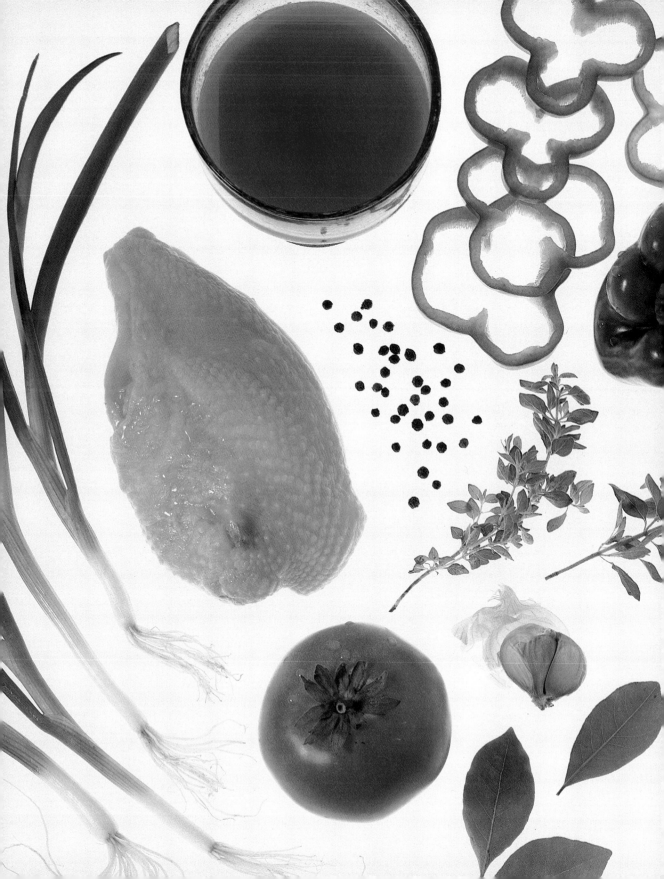

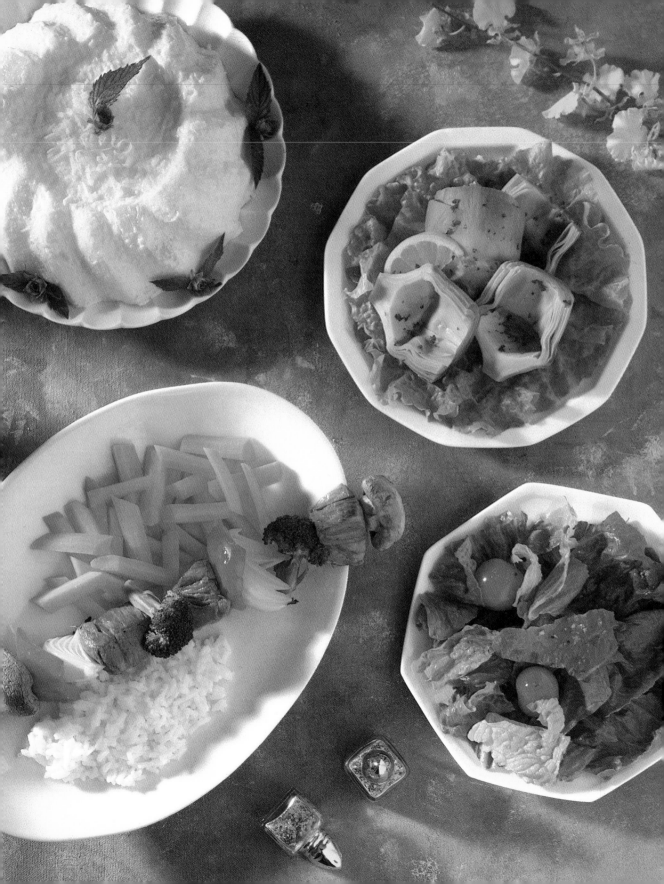

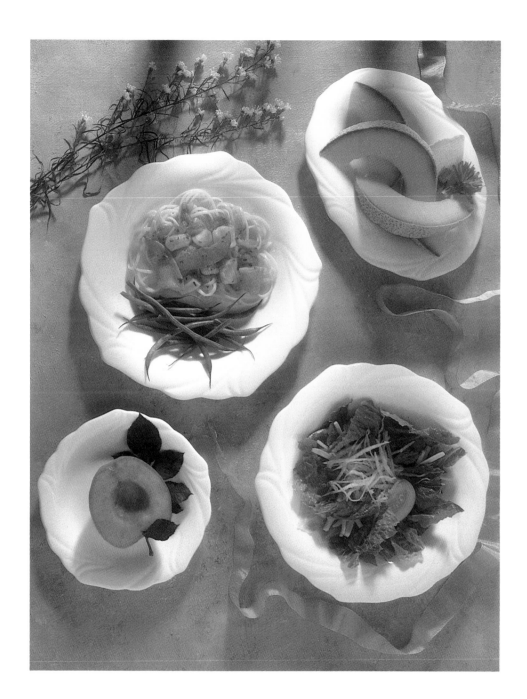

Dinner menu: Melon Slices • Fettuccine with Seafood Marinara • Steamed Green Beans • Garden Salad • Baked Almond Apple *(Photograph by Elizabeth Watt)*

Dinner menu: Artichoke Hearts Vinaigrette • Tenderloin Kabob over Rice • Romaine Salad • Steamed Carrots • Light Cheesecake *(Photograph by Elizabeth Watt)*

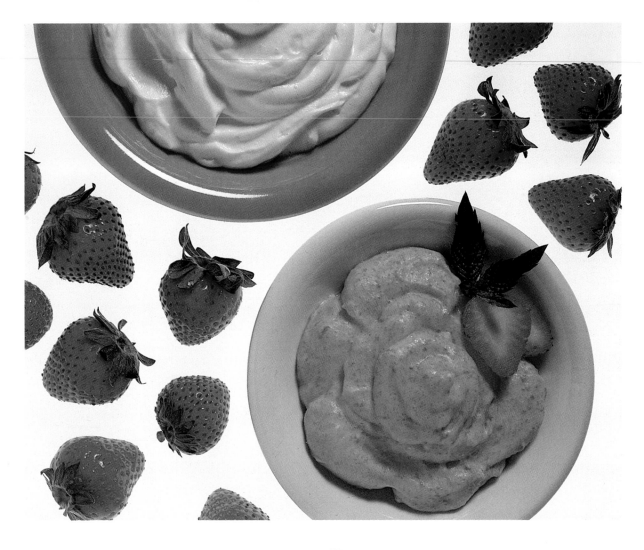

Ingredients for Strawberry Tarts. *(Photograph by Elizabeth Watt)*

Before you begin setting up for your week at home, let's take a moment for a bit of make-believe. Let's see what your schedule would be like if you could escape to Palm-Aire for a week. You may be surprised to see how much of the program you can duplicate at home.

Your Palm-Aire stay would begin with a visit to the doctor to be sure that there were no hidden problems that would make it unwise for you to exercise.

Next you would meet with fitness counselors for tests and measurements to see how you rate right now and to set goals for improvement, both for this week and for the future. Goals go beyond height and weight charts. This is your chance to think about some of the reasons why your life is not the way you would like it to be and what you can do about it, a process that will continue during the week.

The next step is learning how to take your own pulse count to monitor your workouts. The goal is to make the workouts difficult enough to raise your pulse to a target level, but not so strenuous that you will feel exhausted and give up.

Then you are given a personalized schedule that includes exercise and beauty treatments, with the level of exercise determined by your present physical condition.

Late in the day, a film is shown that explains how the Spa regime works. There is an honest warning: You will be sore on day two, tired on day three, and probably cranky as well, wondering whether this is all worthwhile. Day three is the low point. After that the days build to a crescendo by week's end. You begin to feel good all over, discover vitality you may never have experienced before.

Each morning, after a good night's rest, Spa days start off with a delicious breakfast served in your room or in the Spa dining room. A menu might include puffy omelets, a soufflé, or a rich, chewy bran muffin. Almost always there will be delicious fresh fruit, a different kind each morning if you like. Your breakfast beverage is either decaffeinated coffee or an herbal tea, the healthful beverages you will drink all week to cleanse your body of the unnatural effects of caffeine. To make your morning "decaf" more inviting, you may choose to have it flavored with fragrant cinnamon, a taste treat that comes calorie free.

Breakfast includes a multivitamin tablet to ensure you are getting all the nutrients you need during this week of diet and intense activity.

By 9:00 A.M., everyone has assembled at the Spa and is dressed for a brisk 30-minute outdoor walk on the Parcourse. There is a big clock at the beginning of the course, so that you can check your pulse at the start and again after each lap to determine exactly how much exertion it takes to work up to your target pulse rate. By the end of the week you can actually judge how much easier the course seems; your body is able to go farther and move faster.

The day is then divided into alternating periods of exercise and relaxation. For example, 9:40 may bring a class in calisthenics, 10:20 a soak in the whirlpool, and 11:00 A.M. a facial. At 11:40 a spirited water aerobics workout in the pool will leave you refreshed and ready for lunch.

Your nutritious and tempting lunch might be a crisp salad or a surprise treat, perhaps lasagna. The menus have been carefully chosen to include all the food elements a balanced diet requires. If you choose to sit at a group table, while you are enjoying your meal, a member of Palm-Aire's nutrition staff will teach you how to plan equally appealing and healthful menus at home.

The afternoon schedule is much like the morning—at least two exercise sessions, and treatments such as a massage, herbal wrap, or loofah scrub as a reward for your efforts. There is time during the week for a manicure, a pedicure, and consultation on your makeup and hair. Refreshing dips in the big pool or a soothing soak in the whirlpool can be had whenever you need a lift, and Nautilus machines and free weights are available for those who want to add weight training to their schedules. A yoga session is a relaxing and calming way to end the day.

Dinner is a high point—time to enjoy a glass of wine, compare notes with new friends, and marvel once again at how satisfying and imaginative a low-calorie menu can be. More discussions with staff experts are scheduled late in the afternoon and after dinner to enlighten you about stress and how to overcome it and to exchange self-defeating habits for a healthier and happier way of life after you leave the Spa. Said one guest, "As much as I loved all the pleasures and benefited from the workouts, the lectures were the most valuable part of my stay at Palm-Aire. They showed me how it is possible for me to change."

Now it's time for reality. You are ready to learn how to adapt most of this well-rounded program to your own home environment, how to stop procrastinating and set aside one week for shaping up and winding down, just as you would if you were going away to the Spa.

You will see that you can accomplish almost all of the Spa activities at home. You will not be able to devote the same number of hours to exercise while you have personal and professional responsibilities, but an hour and a half a day, divided into half-hour or hour segments, is enough to make a substantial difference, even in a week's time.

You may not have a whirlpool, but a fragrant soak in your own bathtub can still do wonders after exercise and leave you feeling pampered and renewed. Once again, the most important thing is to set aside the time. Part of the luxury of a spa visit is simply having time to concentrate on your own well-being. During this week, you will learn to create this kind of private time for yourself at home. And you will also learn how to make your home feel as special as a spa, with flowers and candles and sweet scents surrounding you everywhere, even in the bath.

In this same pampering spa spirit, you can treat yourself to the few treatments that cannot be duplicated at home by signing up at a local health club, spa, or "Y" for an herbal wrap or full massage in place of one of the home regimens. (If you have a willing partner, you can also follow the instructions on pages 131–32 and learn how to give each other the gift of unequaled relaxation that a skilled massage can bring.)

The delicious Spa menus are a treat at home or away. And if cooking does not seem as glamorous as having meals served to you, remember that there is an important advantage to making these meals for yourself. It is your chance to master the techniques and recipes of spa cuisine that will make weight control far easier for you from now on. You can make these meals feel even more festive by using your best dishes and setting your prettiest table to enjoy them.

The Palm-Aire 7-Day Plan has been carefully devised to provide a pampering week at home that is the next best thing to a spa visit, a week of rejuvenation that is the fresh start you need.

To make the week even more pleasant, you may want to follow the Plan with a spouse or friend, so that you will have some of the moral support that Spa guests often offer one another.

MEASURING UP   Remember that at Palm-Aire, the first step in the week's regimen is a doctor's examination. If you are over forty years old or have not exercised recently, you should see your own physician before you begin this or any other exercise plan.

Then, start your Palm-Aire Plan exactly the way you would at the Spa—record your measurements and set some goals for yourself.

Before you can determine your suggested weight, you must determine your frame size. (See the medium-frame measurement chart that follows.)

Check the height and weight chart to find your suggested weight. As you can see, an ideal weight depends on your age and your body frame. Decide how many pounds you want to lose and set a long-range target date, allowing a loss of no more than two pounds a week. Though you may lose more than that the first week due to the intensity of your exercise and diet combination, in the long run a loss of more than two or three pounds will not be permanent. You will learn why when we talk more about diets in the pages ahead.

MEDIUM-FRAME MEASUREMENTS

Men Height in 1" heels	Elbow Breadth	*Women* Height in 1" heels	Elbow Breadth
5'2"–5'3"	$2\frac{1}{2}$"–$2\frac{7}{8}$"	4'10"–4'11"	$2\frac{1}{4}$"–$2\frac{1}{2}$"
5'4"–5'7"	$2\frac{5}{8}$"–$2\frac{7}{8}$"	5'0"–5'3"	$2\frac{1}{4}$"–$2\frac{1}{2}$"
5'8"–5'11"	$2\frac{3}{4}$"–3"	5'4"–5'7"	$2\frac{3}{8}$"–$2\frac{5}{8}$"
6'0"–6'3"	$2\frac{3}{4}$"–$3\frac{1}{8}$"	5'8"–5'11"	$2\frac{3}{8}$"–$2\frac{5}{8}$"
6'4"	$2\frac{7}{8}$"–$3\frac{1}{4}$"	6'0"	$2\frac{1}{2}$"–$2\frac{3}{4}$"

Source: Copyright © 1983 Metropolitan Life Insurance Company. Source of basic data: 1979 Build Study, Society of Actuaries and Association of Life Insurance Medical Directors of America, 1980.

Note: If your elbow breadth measurement is narrower than the measurement here, you have a small frame. If it is wider, you have a large frame.

MEN

Height Feet Inches		Small Frame	Medium Frame	Large Frame
5	2	128–134	131–141	138–150
5	3	130–136	133–143	140–153
5	4	132–138	135–145	142–156
5	5	134–140	137–148	144–160
5	6	136–142	139–151	146–164
5	7	138–145	142–154	149–168
5	8	140–148	145–157	152–172
5	9	142–151	148–160	155–176
5	10	144–154	151–163	158–180
5	11	146–157	154–166	161–184
6	0	149–160	157–170	164–188
6	1	152–164	160–174	168–192
6	2	155–168	164–178	172–197
6	3	158–172	167–182	176–202
6	4	162–176	171–187	181–207

WOMEN

Height Feet Inches		Small Frame	Medium Frame	Large Frame
4	10	102–111	109–121	118–131
4	11	103–113	111–123	120–134
5	0	104–115	113–126	122–137
5	1	106–118	115–129	125–140
5	2	108–121	118–132	128–143
5	3	111–124	121–135	131–147
5	4	114–127	124–138	134–151
5	5	117–130	127–141	137–155
5	6	120–133	130–144	140–159
5	7	123–136	133–147	143–163
5	8	126–139	136–150	146–167
5	9	129–142	139–153	149–170
5	10	132–145	142–156	152–173
5	11	135–148	145–159	155–176
6	0	138–151	148–162	158–179

Source: Copyright © 1983 Metropolitan Life Insurance Company. Source of basic data: 1979 Build Study, Society of Actuaries and Association of Life Insurance Medical Directors of America, 1980.

Note: Weight in pounds according to frame (in indoor clothing weighing 5 pounds for men and 3 pounds for women; shoes with 1-inch heels).

When you set your goals, remember also that weight is not your only concern. Most of us care far more about how we look than how much we weigh. Muscle tissue weighs more than fat tissue but it is smaller in bulk, firmer, and far more attractive. Since one of your goals is to begin improving your muscle tone through exercise, your looks and measurements can begin to improve even before you lose a number of pounds.

Have someone help you take your measurements for the following chart so that you can keep track of your progress, both in weight and measurements. At the end of the book you will find additional charts to continue marking your progress in the weeks to follow.

PROGRESS REPORT

	First day	Last day	Change
Weight	....	....	....
Neck...............	....	....	....
Upper arm	....	....	....
Forearm	....	....	....
Chest	....	....	....
Bust	....	....	....
Diaphragm........	....	....	....
Waist	....	....	....
Abdomen..........	....	....	....
Hip	....	....	....
Thigh	....	....	....
Calf.................	....	....	....
Knee	....	....	....
Total inches:	....	....	....

A complete fitness analysis goes beyond just body measurements. It also assesses your percentage of body fat, which you hope to reduce, and your strength, flexibility, and cardiovascular condition or endurance, which you hope to increase. Tests you do yourself will not be as accurate as those given by a trained fitness counselor or a doctor, but you can still get a pretty good idea of how you stand with a few simple exercises. Use the tests on pages 11–12 to fill in the chart below, and use it as a record to compare your progress. Don't be discouraged if you don't measure up right now—after all, that's why you are starting a fitness program. The tests are intended to show you where you need work the most.

	Good	Acceptable	Poor
Body fat	....	....	....
Strength	....	....	....
Flexibility	....	....	....
Cardiovascular endurance	....	....	....

BODY FAT: THE PINCH TEST. Your body composition, the ratio of fat to lean muscle tissue, is an important measure that has much to do with your appearance as well as the rate at which your body can burn calories. At Palm-Aire, calipers are used to measure body fat exactly; at home you can get a good idea with your own fingers. Pinch a fold of skin halfway between elbow and shoulder and toward the back of your arm. Then try the same test on top of your hip bone, on your stomach, and on your thigh—the fattest places for most people. A pinch of ¾ to 1 inch is an acceptable range. One-and-a-half inches of fat translates roughly to 30 percent body fat, which means time to shape up!

STRENGTH: THE PUSH-UP TEST. Strength is your muscles' ability to apply force, while endurance measures the muscles' capacity to apply continuous force for a period of time. To do a push-up, lie on the floor face down. Place your hands under your shoulders and straighten your arms to raise your body from the floor, keeping your back straight. To make it a bit easier, place your knees on the floor instead of your feet, bend your legs back at the knee, and cross your feet at the ankles. If you can't do 4 to 6 push-ups, you need to develop your muscle strength. (To build up arm strength, begin by assuming the push-up position, but lower only your body to the floor. With practice you will be able to push up as well.)

FLEXIBILITY: THE FINGERTIP TEST. Sit with your feet placed flat against the wall. Extend your hands until the fingertips touch your toes. If you can't reach them, your flexibility needs improvement.

Another important measure of flexibility involves the hamstring (quadricep) muscles. Many injuries occur when muscles are out of balance. The hamstring, a muscle used whenever we walk, is especially vulnerable. Lie on your back with both knees flexed, arms at your sides. Bring your right knee up as close as possible to your chest and extend your right leg, pointing your toes toward the ceiling. Extend the left leg straight along the floor, so your legs approach a 90-degree angle. Keep your bottom leg and your hip flat on the floor. If you cannot fully extend your raised leg, you need to stretch the hamstring muscles to increase your flexibility.

CARDIOVASCULAR ENDURANCE: YOUR HEART RATE. By monitoring your heart rate, you can determine a safe and effective goal for workouts aimed at increasing your cardiovascular endurance. There are three heart rates to know about in aerobic activities; each of them suggests something about your level of fitness.

Resting Heart Rate (RHR). A person in good aerobic condition usually has a lower resting heart rate than a person in poor condition. The average RHR for women is 78–84; for men it is 72–78. If you are healthy, you may find that as you get involved in aerobic activity, your resting heart rate will go down significantly, indicating that your heart has become stronger. Because it can now pump more blood with each contraction, it does not have to pump as often.

Target Heart Rate (THR). This is the heart rate that indicates the intensity and effectiveness of your workout. As exercise becomes more vigorous, more oxygen is required. The heart increases its rate of beating to supply the needed oxygen and this, in turn, strengthens the heart and promotes aerobic fitness.

Recovery Heart Rate (REHR). This measurement is taken 5 minutes after you've stopped exercising. If your heart rate has not dropped below 120 beats per minute five minutes after you have stopped exercising, you have overextended yourself. Continue walking and stretching until you are below 120. Ten minutes after exercise, the rate should be below 100. If it is not, cut back on the intensity of your workout.

HOW TO TAKE YOUR PULSE

The pulse you feel at your wrist, temple, or carotid artery on either side of your neck is the beat that tells your heart's activity rate. You will need a watch or clock with a second hand to take your pulse. First, monitor your heart at rest. Place your index and middle fingers on the thumb side of your wrist, or at your temple, or place your fingers gently at the carotid artery. Find the beat and count for 10 seconds; then multiply by 6 to get the count for 1 minute. Take a resting heart rate after at least 10 minutes of total inactivity.

Next, you can get an idea of your present level of endurance at home by using a household step stool or the lowest step on a flight of stairs. Step up and down the single step as rapidly as you can for 60 seconds. Now monitor your heart beat again, and compare it with the chart on the following page. Take your Target Heart Rate immediately after you stop exercising because the rate changes very quickly once movement slows or stops.

AVERAGE MAXIMAL HEART RATES AND TARGET ZONES

Age	Maximal	Target Range 70%	85%	Ten-Second Pulse 70%	85%
20	200	140	170	23	28
25	195	137	166	23	28
30	190	133	162	22	27
35	185	130	157	22	26
40	180	126	153	21	26
45	175	123	149	21	25
50	170	119	146	20	24
55	165	116	140	19	23
60	160	112	136	19	23
65	155	109	132	18	22

Source: The Palm-Aire Spa.

As you can see, your heart rate slows with age, and your target rate is adjusted accordingly. Your first goal should be to work up *gradually* during aerobic exercise to 70 percent of your own maximum rate. Remember to check your recovery rate to be sure you are not overdoing it at the start of your 7-Day Spa Plan. This week is not designed to be an endurance test. You are far more likely to stay with your exercise program if you build up slowly rather than exhaust yourself.

Now you should have a set of goals in sight for weight and measurements, and you have determined your weak spots and your cardiovascular targets. You are ready to map out your own 7-Day Plan.

If you follow the plan faithfully, good results are guaranteed. Most important, you will prove to yourself that it is possible to fit an exercise routine and a nutritious diet plan into your present schedule, that you *can* change your ways and follow a healthier life-style.

You will feel and look better at the end of the Palm-Aire 7-Day Plan. And you'll feel a lot better *about* yourself, too.

The Palm-Aire Spa 7-Day Plan

Get ready for a new beginning.

No more excuses, no more "Next week I'm going to get started." Finally you are going to *do* something about your good intentions. You are going to invest 7 days in yourself, 7 days that can change your life.

Those who take a week off to come to the Spa make a sizable investment, demonstrating that taking care of themselves is a priority in their lives. For this week at home, you, too, must declare that taking care of yourself comes first and deserves to be scheduled ahead of everything else.

By acknowledging that your well-being matters, that it is truly worth the investment of time and effort to look and feel better, you have taken the first step toward change.

How are you going to find time for the Palm-Aire Plan in a schedule that already seems overcrowded? It's not as difficult as you think. How to start? Analyze your average day, hour by hour, from the time you wake up in the morning until you go to bed at night. Fill in a practice sheet with the "musts"—work, meal preparation, and any chores or appointments that can't be postponed. Include time for family and friends. Then work with the time spaces left, in half-hour chunks, and fill in the times when it *is* possible for you to exercise and to pamper yourself a bit. When you look for just half an hour at a time, you will find there are many opportunities to gain time for yourself.

What time of day you schedule your Palm-Aire Plan activities does not matter. You can do your thing at 6 A.M. or midnight, use a lunch hour, or set aside free afternoons. For some, it may be easier to scatter free time in 30-minute segments, while others may prefer to combine a number of activities to form one solid block of time. The Palm-Aire home plan is flexible enough to accommodate any daily routine.

A workday schedule may seem inflexible, but with determination you can find the time you need. A full day at the office can accommodate exercise time before and after work and a brisk walk at lunch. Save your pampering for bedtime or schedule a manicure or facial at lunch (and walk there and back!). If necessary, get up 30 minutes earlier each morning. It isn't such an awful prospect if you remember that it's just for this one week. A follow-up plan won't require as much time each day. You may even find that getting started early in the morning is a great way to begin the day.

Those who do not have office hours can schedule their time according to their commitments. Mothers with children in school may want to sandwich most of their activities into the middle of the day when they have the house to themselves, while mothers of infants and toddlers may want to use the time when their children are napping. There are samples on pages 17–23 of a number of ways to plan your days. Whatever your routine, you will discover that exercise has some very practical benefits. Starting the day with exercise sends you off wide awake and bright-eyed in the morning. A brisk walk at lunch will clear your head and make you more productive in the afternoon. You may be surprised to find that rather than making you tired, exercise actually relaxes and energizes you at the end of the day.

Planning your Spa week may also be the catalyst you need to stop procrastinating and enroll in an exercise class or become a member of a health club. Working out with a group can keep you on the track now and encourage you later. If you like, you can also make appointments for a professional facial or massage rather than spend time on beauty treatments at home.

However your schedule falls into place, each day should include the following:

- One *brisk* 30-minute walk
- One 30-minute aerobic workout: biking, swimming, jogging, jumping rope, aerobic dance class, or just steady dancing to lively music at home
- One 30-minute calisthenic exercise routine
- One beauty treatment
- One relaxation technique

Long soaks in the tub are definitely recommended after exercise, whenever time allows. They'll relax you and relieve muscle soreness as well.

Massages are another luxury to be enjoyed whenever you can. Schedule a professional massage or learn with your partner to share this exquisite and healthful pleasure.

Day three is when you are most likely to feel achy and tired from your new regime, so you might want to start the Plan on Friday, and allow time for extra luxurious pampering on Sunday to ease you on to the rest of the week.

Here are some sample days to use as a guide for your own plan. Remember that the menu, exercises, and activities for each day remain the same no matter what time you schedule them.

DAY 1: MONDAY
Sample workday schedule

7 A.M. 30-minute calisthenic routine...
7:30   10 minutes in the tub and dress ....
8:00   Breakfast ....
8:30   Go to work..
9:00   Work ....
9:30   Work ....
10:00   Work ....
10:30   Work ....
11:00   Work ....
11:30   Work ....
12:00   Brisk walk ....
12:30   Lunch...
1:00   Work ....
1:30   Work ....
2:00   Work ....
2:30   Work ....
3:00   Work ....
3:30   Work ....
4:00   Work ....

4:30	Work ....
5:00	Work ....
5:30	Aerobic workout ....
6:15	Shower, prepare dinner ....
7:00	Dinner ....
7:30	Relax ....
8:00	Relax ....
8:30	Relax ....
9:00	Relax ....
9:30	Relax ....
10:00	Treatment: Home facial (see pages 119–20)...........
10:30	Relaxation exercise: Deep Breathing (see page 164)..................
11:00	Bed ....

DAY 2: TUESDAY

Sample stay-at-home schedule

7 A.M.	Brisk walk ....
7:30	Prepare breakfast, get family off...........................
8:00	Prepare breakfast, get family off...........................
8:30	Prepare breakfast, get family off...........................
9:00	Housework ....
9:30	Housework ....
10:00	Housework ....
10:30	Housework ....
11:00	Housework ....
11:30	Exercise ....
12:00	Tub soak ....
12:30	Lunch ....
1:00	Beauty treatment: Manicure (see pages 126–27) ....
1:30	Relaxation technique: Palming (see page 165) ....
2:00	Relaxation technique: Palming ....
2:30	Relaxation technique: Palming ....
3:00	Time with children...
3:30	Time with children...
4:00	Time with children...
4:30	Time with children...
5:00	Time with children...
5:30	Aerobic workout (could be biking or dancing with the kids)........
6:00	Prepare dinner ....
6:30	Dinner ....
7:00	Dinner ....

7:30	Dinner	....
8:00	Clean up	....
8:30	Get children to bed	....
9:00	Relax	....
9:30	Relax	....
10:00	Relax	....
10:30	Relax	....
11:00	Bed	....

DAY 3: WEDNESDAY

Sample workday

7 A.M.	Rise	....
7:30	Shower and dress	....
8:00	Breakfast	....
8:30	Go to work	....
9:00	Work	....
9:30	Work	....
10:00	Work	....
10:30	Work	....
11:00	Work	....
11:30	Work	....
12:00	Brisk walk	....
12:30	Lunch	....
1:00	Work	....
1:30	Work	....
2:00	Work	....
2:30	Work	....
3:00	Work	....
3:30	Work	....
4:00	Work	....
4:30	Work	....
5:00	Get to exercise class	....
5:30	Exercise class	....
6:00	Exercise class	....
6:30	Prepare dinner	....
7:00	Dinner	....
7:30	Dinner	....
8:00	Clean up	....
8:30	Relax	....
9:00	Relax	....
9:30	Aerobic dancing at home	....

10:00   Tub soak: Beauty Treatment: Loofa Scrub (see pages 124–25) ...
10:45   Relaxation technique: Progressive Relaxation (see pages 164–69) ...
11:00   Bed ....

DAY 4: THURSDAY
Sample home day

7 A.M.   Exercise ....
7:30   Shower, dress ....
8:00   Prepare breakfast...
8:30   Get family off ....
9:00   Relax ....
9:30   Housework ....
10:00   Housework ....
10:30   Housework ....
11:00   Brisk walk ....
11:30   Tub soak ....
12:00   Professional or home massage (see pages 129–34).....................
12:30   Lunch..
1:00   Relax ....
1:30   Errands ....
2:00   Committee meeting ....
2:30   Committee meeting ....
3:00   Committee meeting ....
3:30   Time with children...
4:00   Time with children...
4:30   Time with children...
5:00   Time with children...
5:30   Prepare dinner ....
6:00   Dinner ....
6:30   Dinner ....
7:00   Clean up ....
7:30   Relax with family ....
8:00   Relax with family ....
8:30   Relax with family ....
9:00   Children to bed...
9:30   Relax ....
10:00   Relax ....
10:30   Relaxation technique: Relaxing with music (see page 166) ....
11:00   Bed ....

Sample workday

7 A.M.	Rise
7:30	Shower and dress
8:00	Breakfast
8:30	Leave for work
9:00	Work
9:30	Work
10:00	Work
10:30	Work
11:00	Work
11:30	Work
12:00	Lunch
12:30	Brisk walk
1:00	Work
1:30	Work
2:00	Work
2:30	Work
3:00	Work
3:30	Work
4:00	Work
4:30	Work
5:00	Work
5:30	Calisthenics and aerobics workout
6:00	Calisthenics and aerobics workout
6:30	Tub soak
7:00	Beauty treatment: Pedicure (see pages 127–28)
7:15	Relaxation technique: Candle Meditation (see pages 166–67)
7:30	Dress
8:00	Out to dinner
8:30	Out to dinner
9:00	Out to dinner
9:30	Out to dinner
10:00	Out to dinner
10:30	Out to dinner
11:00	Out to dinner
11:30	Bed

Sample schedule

7 A.M.	Rise ....
7:30	....
8:00	Brisk walk ....
8:30	Breakfast ....
9:00	Exercise ....
9:30	Tub soak and dress ....
10:00	....
10:30	Errands ....
11:00	Errands ....
11:30	Errands ....
12:00	Lunch ....
12:30	Lunch ....
1:00	Errands ....
1:30	Errands ....
2:00	Errands ....
2:30	Errands ....
3:00	Relax ....
3:30	Aerobics workout ....
4:00	Tub soak and hair conditioning treatment (see pages 139–40) .....
4:45	Relaxation technique: Visualization (see page 167) ....
5:00	Nap ....
5:30	Nap ....
6:00	Shower, dress for evening out ....
6:30	Shower, dress for evening out ....
7:00	Evening out ....
7:30	Evening out ....
8:00	Evening out ....
8:30	Evening out ....
9:00	Evening out ....
9:30	Evening out ....
10:00	Evening out ....
10:30	Evening out ....
11:00	Evening out ....
11:30	Bed ....

DAY 7: SUNDAY
Sample schedule

7 A.M.	Rise..
7:30	....
8:00	....
8:30	....
9:00	Aerobic exercise..
9:30	Breakfast..
10:00	....
10:30	Relax..
11:00	Relax..
11:30	Relax..
12:00	Relax..
12:30	Prepare lunch...
1:00	Lunch..
1:30	Lunch..
2:00	Beauty treatment: Facial (see pages 119–23).................
2:30	Experiment with makeup preparations (see pages 135–38)......
3:00	Relax with family, friends..................................
3:30	Relax with family, friends..................................
4:00	Relax with family, friends..................................
4:30	Relax with family, friends..................................
5:00	Exercise..
5:30	Relaxation technique: Yoga (see pages 167–69)..............
6:00	Tub soak..
6:15	Prepare dinner..
7:00	Dinner..
7:30	Brisk walk..
8:00	Evening free to relax.......................................
8:30	Evening free to relax.......................................
9:00	Evening free to relax.......................................
9:30	Evening free to relax.......................................
10:00	Evening free to relax.......................................
10:30	Evening free to relax.......................................
11:00	Bed...

So there you have it—a variety of workable schedules for a full week of renewal for your body and your mind.

Only one thing remains to be done before you are ready to begin: You have to prepare a shopping list. You should have all the menu ingredients and beauty preparations you need on hand in advance so that you can carry out the parts of your Plan easily and without delays. Check the menu section and make out a grocery shopping list. You will find you probably have the basic ingredients needed for many menus, but it is important to read through and shop ahead so that your recipe will not be ruined for lack of an essential ingredient.

Use the following checklist as your guide to the other things you will need. Many of these are common household items and cosmetics that you normally have on hand, but some may require a special shopping expedition.

Have fun while you shop for your week of beauty and exercise—make it a time to indulge in some new scents for your bath, select new colors for your makeup or nails. Treat yourself to an exercise mat or a new makeup mirror along with the essentials. Buy a bright new leotard or workout shorts, knowing you are going to look better in them with every passing day!

Note: Some of the items for your face, listed below, can be made from natural ingredients in your refrigerator or cupboards. See "Making the Most of Yourself" on beauty for details.

PALM-AIRE PLAN SHOPPING CHECKLIST

For your face
Milk-type facial cleanser
Large roll of cotton
Skin toner
Moisturizer
Lubricating cream
Cleansing granules
Facial mask
Eye cream
Eye makeup remover
Headband or hair clips
Magnifying makeup mirror

For your hair
Natural bristle brush
Protein pack or conditioning treatment

For your body
Body lotion
Bath lotion
Natural body oils
Loofah scrub mitt
Kosher salt

24

For manicures and pedicures

Emery boards

Orangewood sticks

Cotton

Polish remover

Cuticle cream

Mild soap

Cotton swabs

Nail polish

Base and top coats

Hand cream

Pumice stone

While you are checking the requirements for the week, don't forget one of the prime targets of the Palm-Aire Plan—your morale. Reward yourself with luxury this week. Some of the following things can help make you feel really special:

Scented soap
Bubble bath
Fluffy new towels and robe
Fresh after-bath cologne
New waterproof radio for shower and/or bath
New shades of makeup and nail polish
New exercise outfits
A pretty atomizer for your dresser to hold cologne or distilled water
Potpourri to scent your rooms
Fresh flowers to lift your spirits
Sparkling wine—or Champagne—to toast a successful end to the week!

Along with equipping yourself with these essential tools (and goodies), you will need some equally essential information. The chapters ahead will provide all the techniques you need for exercise, nutritious menu planning, stress reduction, and beauty treatments, plus seven days worth of delicious low-calorie recipes. They will help you understand how your body works so you can help it function better. They will point out to you some of the difficulties that may have kept you from a healthier life-style in the past, and teach you how to exchange old habits and patterns for better new ones.

The information here, adapted from lectures given at Palm-Aire, is aimed at helping you achieve not just weight loss but the true fitness and sense of well-being that will give you new energy and optimism—and help you to find a new outlook that can change your life.

Shaping-Up: What You Need to Know

If you are going to succeed with this or any shape-up plan, there are some important things you should know about how and why your body reacts to diet and exercise.

Most of us have a lot of misconceptions about what it takes to get ourselves into shape. One of the things most people know least about, in fact, is the very thing that bothers them most: body fat. The way most people change their diets in an attempt to lose weight is the surest way *not* to lose that unwanted fat. Here are three facts that you must understand if you want to reduce body fat.

FACT 1: *Losing weight is not the same thing as losing fat.*

FACT 2: *Going on a crash diet can be the surest way to gain both weight and fat.*

FACT 3: *Speeding up the way your body metabolizes or burns fat is the only path to permanent weight loss.*

Here's why. Your body is made up of two kinds of tissue: fat and lean. Lean tissue, or muscle, is not only more attractive, but burns calories faster than fatty tissue does. The body needs a certain amount of reserve fat tissue for warmth and as a source of extra energy, so it hoards fat, using it up slowly. Excess fat is burned at the same slow rate as that necessary reserve of fat. The greater the percentage of your excess fat compared to lean tissue, the slower is your metabolism—the rate at which the body uses calories. That's why it can be sad but true that you and your skinniest best friend can eat identical servings of pie à la mode, but the bulges will show only on *your* frame. It hardly seems fair, but a lean frame simply burns calories more efficiently.

Now that you know that excess fat is the culprit, you realize that your goal in shaping-up is not simply to lose pounds, especially not to lose the healthy lean tissue that works so efficiently. To change the way your body functions, you must reduce the percentage of fat tissue to lean tissue, because excess fat not only creates unsightly bulges but actually makes it more difficult for you to lose weight by slowing down the metabolism.

In other words, losing pounds is not enough: You need to lose *fat*— and dieting alone cannot do that.

First of all, when you diet without exercising at the same time to strengthen your muscles, at least a third of the weight lost comes off the muscles, that lean tissue you don't want to lose.

Second, as soon as you go back to old eating habits, any weight lost will come back—and it *all* comes back as fat. The more drastic the diet, the faster you may gain afterward. That's because your body's calorie-burning mechanism sets itself according to the number of calories it receives. Your metabolism is used to operating on your normal food intake. When you diet, cutting down on the calories coming in, your body adjusts to the shortage by conserving energy, burning fewer calories than usual. You might compare it to having to live off your savings account rather than your checking account for a while. The natural reaction is to spend less.

It is this slowed metabolism that makes it harder to lose weight after about the first week of a stringent diet. The body simply adjusts to getting along on less by slowing things down.

After you go off a diet and begin taking in additional calories, the metabolism doesn't swing right back to its old set point. It remains for quite a while at the slower metabolic rate until it gets the message to speed up again. So the additional calories you are now consuming will not be used up, but stored up—as extra fat. Each time you go on and off a diet, you first lose some muscle tissue while you eat less and then add extra fat tissue once you resume your old eating habits. The percentage of fat to lean actually increases so that you are fatter than when you started. You have added more fat tissue, which burns calories so inefficiently.

Equally harmful, each time you diet unsuccessfully, is that you are likely to become further discouraged about your ability to lose weight. You blame it on lack of willpower, and you don't like yourself. A typical reaction is to bury your sorrow in food! After all, if dieting doesn't work anyway, why not at least enjoy eating?

How to break this vicious cycle? The first step is to avoid drastic start-and-stop dieting. Stop starving yourself. It only slows down your body's ability to burn calories. Aim instead to take weight off gradually and steadily. In the next chapter, you'll read more about the Palm-Aire eating strategy. It shows you the type of menus you can follow for life, not just for a week or two.

The next step is to begin modifying your body composition, changing the percentage of fat to lean so that your overall metabolism will work faster all the time, helping you continue to lose weight.

Instead of slowing down your metabolism with crazy diets, your goal is to *speed it up*—to build muscle and get rid of fat. In other words, to become *fit* instead of fat.

THINKING FIT

Fitness is another word we hear often, but don't always understand properly. To an athlete, fitness may mean training in order to perform better. To someone with high blood pressure, fitness may be the key to cardio-vascular health and a longer life.

For anyone who wants to lose weight, fitness has still another meaning: getting the body's metabolism working so that it will use more calories and speed weight loss now. It also means building the ratio of muscle to fat, enabling the body to metabolize more and more efficiently as time goes on.

The best way to accomplish this is with the kind of exercises called *aerobic*. Aerobic exercises, such as jogging, brisk walking, skipping rope, biking, or swimming, are those in which the body utilizes a lot of oxygen to produce energy. They are exercises using the large muscles of the body in a sustained, intense effort that increases the heart rate and literally causes you to breathe harder, drawing in more oxygen. The body needs the oxygen to manufacture the extra fuel you need to keep going at an increased heart rate. It makes this fuel by combining the oxygen intake with fatty acids from the body's stored fat. While all exercise that moves the muscles aids in metabolizing fat, aerobics are the most efficient way to metabolize the greatest amount of fat in the least amount of time.

When muscles work, they first call on glycogen, a source of short-term energy contained in the muscles themselves. After about 12 minutes of aerobic exercise, the body hears the call for extra energy that cannot be met by glycogen alone, and begins metabolizing fat to get it. After 20 minutes, it reaches its most efficient energy-burning capacity. Equally important, after a 20- to 30-minute aerobic workout, your metabolic rate *remains* elevated for as long as 5 to 15 hours. That means if you work out in the morning, the body will be burning calories faster for most of the day.

And the benefits grow the longer you continue an aerobic program of exercise. Aerobically conditioned muscle actually changes its biochemical structure in order to utilize oxygen more efficiently and, therefore, continually burns calories at a higher rate. You cannot swap fat for muscle, but through aerobics you can reduce the percentage of fat in your body compared to the percentage of muscle. And you will be on the way to becoming *metabolically slender,* changing the way your body operates, so it uses more calories regularly.

Calorie-burning aerobics are also your best bet for removing those fatty bulges from thighs or stomach, because there is really no such thing as "spot reducing." You may tone and firm muscles with calisthenics or weight training, but you need aerobic exercise to reduce fatty deposits most effectively. Over a period of time, aerobics will burn up excess fat, proportionately, throughout the entire body.

Aerobics offer other benefits as well in the form of increased cardiovascular endurance, which means a stronger and more efficiently operating heart. Sustained exercise is also a proven stress reducer. New research indicates that increased oxygen to the brain through a steady aerobics program may even improve the memory. And if you need any further persuasion that aerobics should be a part of your life, it's a happy fact that the more energy you put out in aerobic exercise, the more energy you get back to see you through the other activities in your life. The more you exercise, the less tired you will feel!

Now you understand why the Palm-Aire Plan stresses aerobics—a brisk walk and a good workout daily. Try a number of kinds of aerobics this week and find the ones you like and believe you can stay with. If you hate to jog, don't—dance, instead, or ride a bike. You will find a number of suggestions for aerobic activities in the chapter on shaping up.

One misconception, discouraging some people from trying aerobics, is the idea that they are tremendously hard work. Happily, you don't have to go all out in order for exercise to produce results. It is best to start slowly and build a bit more endurance each day, without exhausting yourself. Becoming fit takes time; but you don't have to rush it. You will not have to wait until you have met your final fitness goals to lose weight.

LSD (Long Slow Distance) is the key to weight loss. It takes the same amount of energy to move a weight slowly over a given distance as to move it quickly. That means you will burn as many calories walking briskly for a mile as running for a mile. It's the total distance and the steady time you invest that counts.

And, as we have seen, calories are not the whole story. With aerobics you are changing your body chemistry, not just taking off a quick pound or two. In the long run, you will really lose pounds—and they will stay off.

So don't strain and burn out trying to do too much right away. Just start moving and you will begin to burn calories. *Gradually* increase your pulse rate and you will increase your aerobic capacity as well. At the end of just one week, you will see that you can do more without strain, and you will have already established a pattern of exercise that can fit into your schedule and become a constant in your life.

Meanwhile, your changes of habit should extend into the kitchen. Together with exercise, carefully balanced menus and adherence to a sensible, low-calorie food plan is the secret to *true* weight loss—not the false loss of fad diets.

A moderate diet combined with exercise is the speediest way to achieve permanent weight loss.

Diet only
Cutting 500 calories per day for seven days equals 1 pound lost (70 percent fat, 30 percent lean).

Exercise only
Jogging 3 times a week equals ½ pound lost (mostly fat).

Diet and exercise
Moderate diet and exercise equals 1½ pounds lost plus more muscle tissue built, which lowers the percentage of body fat even more than the weight loss indicates.

- Dieting alone is the *least* effective way to lose fat.
- When the scale says you have lost weight, that does not always mean a loss of fat. In the first week of a fad diet, usually up to 70 percent of the weight loss is water depletion. Any low-calorie diet that creates a weight loss over 2 pounds per week is temporarily reducing water rather than permanently reducing fat. The loss won't last!
- Fad dieting makes it easier to gain weight on less food. When you reduce the number of calories you take in, your body activates its "survival" mechanism, slowing down the metabolism to adjust to a lower caloric intake. It simply learns to function on less fuel, using up fewer calories to do the same amount of work. If you lose weight by strict dieting and then go back to normal eating without adding exercise, you will regain the original weight *plus* added pounds, because a metabolism slowed to meet diet calorie intake will not be able to burn calories at its old normal level when you begin eating normally again.
- The pounds regained when you go off a crash diet are all fat. They may actually increase the percentage of fat in your body while the percentage of muscle remains constant or decreases; therefore, you may be more obese than before you started.
- Calisthenic or "anaerobic" exercise tones and builds muscle, which weigh more than fat. However, muscle takes up less space than fat. Your measurements may change and you may look better, but you will *not* be losing weight.
- Aerobic exercise is the exercise that metabolizes fat most efficiently; the body draws upon fat for sustained energy to move the muscles and to help the heart remain in a target zone for 20 minutes.
- The combination of aerobic exercise and a sound diet is the most effective weight-loss/inch-loss program.

The Palm-Aire Exercise Book

"Please don't give in to the common thinking that sagging muscles, poor posture, back pains, and double chins are part of life . . . or simply 'old age creeping up.'

"The truth is that your muscles, through improper or lack of use, cause these bulges and pains. Also, through your muscles, nature has given you the means to preserve good health and good looks throughout life."

So reads a message on the body measurement chart given to guests at Palm-Aire. It is a fitting introduction to an exercise guide because correct exercise is the key to fitness that will restore muscle tone, improve your appearance, and boost your vitality no matter what your age.

Unless you do something to counteract the slowing metabolism that comes with age, it is possible to lose a little muscle tone and put on a depressing pound of weight every year after the age of twenty-five. Calorie-counting and regular exercise are the only antidotes. Being a movie star or a celebrity doesn't exempt you from nature's laws; evidence of this are the many fitness-conscious stars who frequent the Palm-Aire Spa to keep themselves in tip-top shape.

Your own Palm-Aire Plan week at home is a big step in the right direction. To make sure it's a plan you'll stay with long enough to see long-term results, begin slowly and build up gradually; don't push yourself to your limit at the start. Remember that fitness and performance are not the same thing. Most of us are not athletes competing for Olympic medals. The rewards we seek are personal—the self-confidence and pride that comes with a trimmer, more agile body and the increased energy level and zest for life that regular exercise produces. These are long-term goals. Going all out at a pace you can't maintain will only leave you sore and exhausted, not raring to go—and keep going. So rather than push to see how much you can do, aim for a steady, enjoyable level that will encourage you to continue in the weeks ahead.

Remember, too, that there is no "best exercise." The most effective exercises for you are simply the ones you are most likely to stick with.

At the Spa, almost every guest finds some exercises that have more appeal for them than others. Elizabeth Taylor enjoyed doing water aerobics exercises with a kick board, while Liza Minnelli liked working out on the stationary bike. Mary Tyler Moore was enthusiastic about the new controlled-impact aerobic dance classes, and both she and her husband appreciated the relaxation of yoga.

A well-rounded exercise plan stresses aerobics, which includes walking, but also incorporates calisthenics for strengthening and toning the muscles, and stretching exercises for flexibility. Palm-Aire's special routines are in the pages ahead. Water exercises offer a double bonus—pressure that makes each exercise more effective plus cushioning that eases stress on the joints. Ninety percent of your body weight is displaced in water.

Sociable sports, such as skiing, tennis, and golf, do not take the place of aerobic workouts, but they are good exercise and calorie-burners.

How many calories you burn in sports and exercise depends on your weight and the intensity of your activity. The more you weigh, the more calories your body must use to move around, and obviously, it takes more energy for a fast game of tennis singles than for a leisurely mixed doubles match. A 60-minute stroll at 2 miles an hour costs a 120-pound person 165 calories, while a brisker pace of 3.5 miles an hour would use 280 calories.

Here is a chart to show you the calories used for various activities at different weights:

ENERGY EXPENDITURES IN VARIOUS ACTIVITIES

	Calories per minute per your weight in pounds				
	100	120	140	170	200
Badminton-recreation	4.3	5.2	6.1	7.4	8.7
Basketball-moderate	4.6	5.6	6.5	7.9	9.3
Bicycling 5.5 mph	3.1	3.8	4.4	5.3	6.3
Bicycling 10 mph	5.4	6.5	7.6	9.2	10.8
Bowling nonstop	4.4	5.3	6.2	7.5	8.8
Calisthenics	3.3	3.9	4.6	5.6	6.6
Canoeing 2.5 mph	1.9	2.3	2.7	3.3	3.9
Canoeing 4.0 mph	4.6	5.6	6.5	7.9	9.3
Mod dance (moderate)	2.7	3.3	3.8	4.7	5.5
Mod dance (vigorous)	3.7	4.5	5.2	6.4	7.5
Golf	3.6	4.3	5.0	6.1	7.2
Handball	6.3	7.6	8.8	10.7	12.7
Judo, karate (cont.)	8.6	10.3	12.0	14.6	17.2

Mountain climbing	6.6	8.0	9.3	11.3	13.3
Jogging 11-min. mile	6.1	7.3	8.5	10.4	12.2
Jogging 8-min. mile	9.4	11.3	13.2	16.0	18.8
Jogging 7-min. mile	10.2	12.2	14.2	17.3	20.4
Jogging 5-min. mile	13.1	15.7	18.4	22.3	26.3
Racquetball	6.3	7.6	8.8	10.7	12.7
Rowing (machine)	8.1	9.7	11.4	13.8	16.3
Running in place	9.5	11.4	13.3	16.1	19.0
Skating (moderate)	3.6	4.3	5.0	6.1	7.2
Skiing downhill	6.3	7.6	8.8	10.7	12.7
Skiing cross-country	7.2	8.7	10.1	12.3	14.5
Snowshoeing 2.5 mph	5.8	7.0	8.2	10.0	11.7
Squash	6.8	8.1	9.5	11.5	13.6
Swimming backstroke	4.5	5.4	6.3	7.7	9.0
Swimming breaststroke	4.8	5.7	6.7	8.1	9.6
Swimming crawl	5.8	6.9	8.1	9.8	11.6
Table tennis	2.7	3.2	3.8	4.6	5.4
Tennis (recreation)	4.5	5.4	6.4	7.7	9.1
Volleyball (moderate)	2.3	2.7	3.2	3.9	4.6
Walking 2.0 mph	2.2	2.7	3.1	3.8	4.5
Walking 3.0 mph	2.7	3.2	3.8	4.6	5.4
Walking 4.0 mph	3.9	4.6	5.4	6.6	7.8
Weight training (cont.)	4.9	5.9	6.9	8.4	9.9

Source: The Complete Book of Physical Fitness by A. Garth Fisher and Robert K. Conlee, Brigham Young Press, Provo, Utah, 1979. Adapted from C. Frank Consolazio, Robert E. Johnson, and Louis J. Perora. *Physiological Measurements of Metabolic Functions in Man*, McGraw-Hill Book Co., New York, 1963, and from data developed at the Human Performance Research Center at Brigham Young University, Provo, Utah.

Whatever kind of exercise you do, always include a warm-up and a cool-down period. Neither your muscles nor your heart should be expected to shift into high gear without any warning. Just as you would ease your car from neutral to progressively higher gears, you should warm up your body to protect it from sprains or strains. It is equally important to cool down after exercising. When you exercise, a lot of blood is sent to the legs to keep the large muscles adequately supplied with oxygen. While the legs are moving, that blood is helped back to the heart by the squeezing action of the muscles. If you stop suddenly, cutting off the muscle movement, the heart and brain may experience a temporary shortage of blood, resulting in lightheadedness, dizziness, or nausea. The reason marathon runners continue walking after an exhausting race is to avoid that kind of reaction.

What is the best time for exercise? The time you are most likely to do it. Once again, this week is your chance to experiment. See how you can best fit periods of exercise into your normal day.

PALM-AIRE EXERCISE DO'S AND DON'TS

You will get the most benefit from exercise with the least strain if you follow these guidelines:

1. If you have been sedentary and are just beginning an exercise program, start slowly. Attempting a "gung-ho" approach at first only leads to exhaustion and discouragement.

2. If you feel fatigued, slow down your pace, but do *not* stop exercising. Keep moving, no matter how little.

3. Follow your own exercise goals—don't try to keep up with others. Your goals should be personal.

4. If you exceed your target heart rate range, slow down.

5. Never go immediately from a sitting or reclining position to a high level of activity or from vigorous activity to a resting state. Work your tempo up and down gradually. Allow 5 to 10 minutes for warm-up activity before a workout and 3 to 5 minutes for rhythmic cool-down exercises at the end.

6. Five minutes after you finish exercising, check your recovery heart rate. If the rate is more than 120, you are doing too much. Cut down either the intensity or the length of your workout.

7. Exercises such as weight lifting or isometrics build muscular strength and calisthenics tone the muscles, but they do little to promote cardiovascular fitness. These activities should be done in conjunction with a regular program of aerobic exercise.

8. Do not expect instant results. You will see progress from an introductory week of steady workouts, but it will not last unless you continue to exercise. Sustained improvements in fitness levels begin after 1 to 2 months of an exercise program and increase further during the following months.

9. Try to exercise every other day, not allowing more than 48 hours to pass between workouts. Brisk walks definitely count. If every other day

is not possible, a minimum of 3 times a week has been shown to result in significant improvement in cardiovascular fitness.

PALM-AIRE EXERCISE CAUTIONS

1. Never perform exercises that involve bouncing, rapid change of direction, or locking or hyperextending a joint.

2. If you are inactive for 2 weeks or more, do not resume your exercise program at the point where you left off. Allow at least as much time as you took off to work back up to your former level.

3. Avoid the following exercises, which may put strain on the back:
   double leg lifts (raising and lowering both legs simultaneously from a
   reclining position)
   sit-ups with straight legs
   standing toe touches
   back bends.

4. Avoid deep knee bends to prevent injury to the knee joint.

5. If you have knee problems, omit exercises that put pressure on your knees or are done on your hands and knees.

6. If you have not exercised recently or are over the age of forty, have a medical checkup before you begin any exercise regimen.

AEROBIC EXERCISE

Calorie-burning aerobics are the key to steady weight loss—and to strengthening your heart. Aerobics means any brisk exercise that uses the body's large muscles and lasts long enough to require extra oxygen as energy to keep those muscles going. The body calls on stored fat, which metabolizes in the presence of oxygen to produce long-term muscle energy. This is why energy-intense aerobics are the most efficient way to get rid of fat. Aerobically conditioned muscle also changes its biochemical structure eventually in order to use oxygen more efficiently and begins to use calories at a higher rate for all your daily activities, helping you further to control your weight.

Aerobic exercise has other benefits as well. Besides building cardiovascular endurance, it strengthens muscles and bones, increases energy, and reduces stress. Many people find it also reduces the appetite.

The formula to gain these many benefits is an easy one to remember. Just think of FIT:

F = frequency. Exercise at least 3 times per week, preferably every other day.
I = intensity. Exercise hard enough to raise your heart rate to 70 to 85 percent of your maximum heart rate. (MHR = 220 minus your age; see page 13.)
T = time. Keep your heart rate within the target level for 20 to 40 minutes.

There are many kinds of aerobic exercises, each with some advantages and disadvantages, so try several and find the ones you most enjoy. Persistence at one kind of exercise helps you to build endurance and become better at it, but you don't have to stick to one kind of activity if it becomes boring. Better to vary your aerobics and keep at them!

Remember, to have cardiovascular and weight-control value, the exercise must be performed at your Target Heart Rate for a minimum of 20 minutes at least 3 to 4 times a week. Here are some of the aerobic conditioners to choose from.

WALKING

The easiest, safest, and most overlooked aerobic exercise of all, walking is an enjoyable and beneficial exercise. When weather prevents walking outside, indoor tracks or treadmill walking can be substituted. You can elevate your heart rate in various ways as you walk:

1. Increase speed and swing arms vigorously

2. Carry light weights (1 to 2 pounds) in your hands

3. Walk in hilly terrain

4. On a treadmill, increase the incline rather than the speed

JOGGING/RUNNING

This is an excellent aerobic activity and a proven stress reducer. But it takes time to work into condition to be able to jog for the required 20 to 40 minutes, and jogging sometimes takes a toll on hips, knees, or ankles. At the start, try alternating jogging and walking to build up endurance. Like walking, jogging can be done on a treadmill or indoor track in bad weather.

BICYCLING

Cycling programs put less pressure on the joints than an exercise such as jogging, and they are versatile, since a stationary bicycle can substitute for bicycling out of doors when the weather is inclement. Some exercise bikes also come with arm levers for an even more complete body work-out. Outdoor bicycling is one of the most pleasant ways to exercise, but to be beneficial, remember that it should be done away from traffic that requires frequent stops. The exercise must be continuous to be aerobic.

SWIMMING

Swimming has the distinct advantage of using the upper as well as the lower body. The water supplies a cushioning effect that is helpful to the joints. It also dissipates body heat generated by exercise, making you more comfortable while you exercise. It is especially recommended for those who are very overweight. The one drawback is that you must master a basic stroke in order to have a true aerobic workout. Just paddling or floating around is not enough. If swimming interests you but you don't swim well, you might consider taking lessons. You can also learn a water aerobics exercise regimen that will provide a good workout in only four feet of water.

STAIR CLIMBING/STEPPING

Another often overlooked activity, stepping is excellent for the beginner or an obese person because the foot is placed flat on the stair using the large leg muscles and eliminating unnecessary pressure on the joints. You can use an existing set of stairs or a single wooden box between 8 and 15 inches high. Just step up one foot at a time and then back down to the floor. A number of combinations of foot and arm work can be used to vary the exercise. Then try flights of stairs.

REBOUNDING

Jogging, jumping, skipping, hopping, and bouncing are some of the move-ment patterns that can be performed on a minitrampoline or rebounder. This is an exercise that feels much like play, and the trampoline cushions the shock on the joint areas. It may take a few tries to get used to the equilibrium required, but many people find this an enjoyable way to ex-ercise.

JUMPING ROPE

Elevating the heart rate while jumping rope is easy for most people. The problem is that the calf muscles do most of the work and usually fatigue quickly, making it hard to keep going. A program of rope jumping sup-plemented by walking or jogging can be a good combination. Alternate the activities to fill out a 20- to 40-minute exercise period.

INDOOR/OUTDOOR ROWING

Rowing is an excellent total body aerobic activity using the large muscles of the back as well as the large leg muscles. Most indoor rowing machines are equipped with variable resistance levels so that you can set the machine to your own individual fitness level.

AEROBIC DANCE

One of the most popular forms of aerobic activity, aerobic dance is spirited fun, but in order to be truly aerobic, you must make sure the dance steps are done at an appropriate intensity. Use a watch or clock with a second hand to check your pulse rate every 10 minutes during your exercise period, making sure you are at the target level. If you take a class, remember that music sometimes masks the intensity of the dance, and take care not to overdo. At home, all you have to do for an aerobic workout is to put on lively music and keep moving to the beat.

Aerobic dance does have one possible drawback because constant jumping and bouncing can stress the joints. If you have problems with your knees or just find the pace of regular aerobic dancing too strenuous, try Palm-Aire's controlled-impact aerobic workout. The only difference is that there is no jumping and one foot remains on the floor at all times. They still get your pulse going to fast-stepping music, but are much easier on the body.

Music is all important in aerobics. It should inspire you to keep moving. You can choose your own favorite records—Bach or Basie, bluegrass or rock—just as long as the beat is brisk. If you prefer, most record stores now stock music especially designed for aerobic workouts. Many exercise studios also subscribe to a quarterly publication called *The Aerobic Beat* (Ken Alan Associates, 7985 Santa Monica Blvd., Suite 109, Los Angeles, CA 90046). It lists an aerobic "Top 30" in each issue, the music that is most popular in aerobic dance programs around the country, and includes currently popular music suggestions for warm-up and calisthenic workouts as well. If you plan to make dancing your main aerobic exercise, you might want to subscribe in order to vary the music and keep things more interesting.

Begin with a moderate tempo for warm-ups; then work up progressively to a faster beat. Your pulse check will tell you whether you need a quicker tempo.

Common aerobic dance steps include jogging in place, skipping, hopping, marching, knee lifts, forward and backward kicks, jumps, and twists, combined with up-and-down and pushing-and-pulling arm movements. Many of the arm movements are the same as calisthenic exercises and help to tone the muscles at the same time you are getting an aerobic workout.

40

One suggested aerobic dance routine follows. It is hard to follow printed instructions and keep up a dance pace, so become familiar with the steps and routines before you begin. Once you get the basics, you can easily improvise with your own routines. As the workout becomes easier, you can make it more demanding by adding hand and ankle weights. Always remember to drop the heel while running in place so that the calves do not tighten.

30-Minute Aerobic Dance Workout

WARM-UP: 5 *MINUTES*

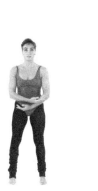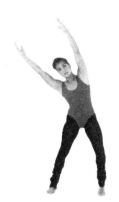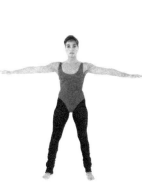

1. Stand with your feet slightly apart and your arms at your sides. Inhale as you lift your arms up to the ceiling; stretch high and exhale as you swing your arms back down to cross in front of your body. Repeat 3 times.

2. Lift your arms to the ceiling and stretch over to the side. Alternate left and right stretches, lifting the opposite heel on each stretch. Repeat 6 times, alternating direction.

3. Hold your arms straight out to the side at shoulder height. Point your fingers out and stretch toward the opposite walls, first right and then left, moving only the top half of your body. Repeat 8 times in each direction.

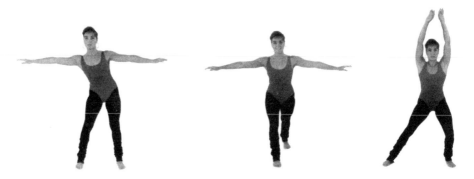

4. Repeat the side to side movement, rotating your palms face up and down with each stretch. Repeat 8 times in each direction.

5. With your arms still outstretched at shoulder level, bend your left knee and lunge forward, to the left. Straighten and lunge to the right. Alternate from side to side, 8 times in each direction.

6. Repeat the lunges from left to right, lifting your opposite arms up to the ceiling as you bend, 8 times in each direction.

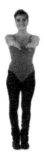 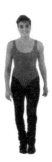

7. Repeat the lunges, swinging both of your arms up and down in the direction of the lunge, 8 times in each direction.

8. Step-touch from side to side, moving your left foot to the right and then your right foot to the left, swinging both of your arms out in front of your body in the direction of the step, and keeping your elbows close to your body, 4 times in each direction.

9. Step in place, lifting your heels only, swinging your arms gently, 8 times, alternating left to right.

10. Continue stepping in place, raising your arms up to the ceiling and back down to your sides with each step. Repeat 16 times.

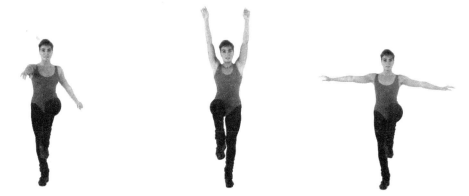

Change to music with a faster tempo.

1. March in place briskly, knees high and arms swinging, 16 times.

2. Keep marching, swinging your arms all the way overhead and all the way back, 16 times.

3. Hold your arms out to the sides; lift your left knee to your chest; then lift your right knee, each side 8 times.

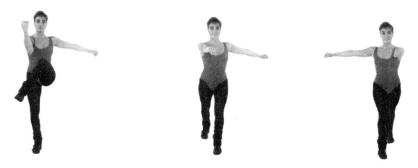

4. Continue lifting your knees, and extend your right elbow to meet your left knee as it comes up; then do the same with your left elbow to your right knee, each side 12 times.

5. Step forward with your left foot and punch hard to the left with your right hand; then step forward with your right foot and punch to the right with your left hand, 4 times each way. Follow by punching straight up overhead, alternating hands, each side 4 times; then punch across in front of your chest, again alternating sides, 4 times each side.

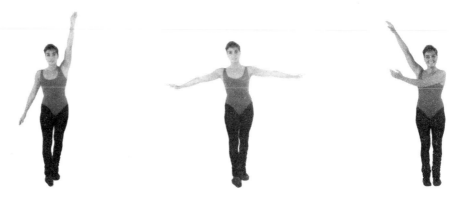

6. Do an easy toe-heel motion alternating feet, lifting your right arm toward the ceiling 8 times, then your left arm 8 times, then both arms 16 times

7. Continuing toe and heel motion, briskly lift your arms up high and down 2 times and then out to the sides at shoulder height 2 times and down 2 times.

8. Do 4 quick side steps to the right in time to the music, swinging your arms up as you go. Repeat to the left, 8 times in each direction.

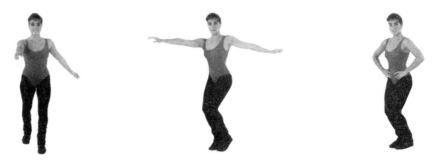

9. Take 4 steps forward to the beat of the music, swinging your arms back and forth; then take 4 steps back, 12 times in each direction.

10. Using the balls of your feet as a pivot, shift your heels from side to side, twisting your body from the waist down 8 times; lift your arms to the ceiling and repeat 8 twists.

11. Pony step (right foot, left foot, right foot) to the right and then to the left, 4 times each way. Repeat, lifting your arms overhead to alternating sides as you step.

12. Take 4 brisk steps forward in time to the music; then go back to place, swinging your arms as you go, 12 times each way.

13. Pony step again, forward and back this time, arms also swinging forward and back, 8 times each way.

14. Bounce lightly in place 8 times; then bounce and twist at the same time 8 times.

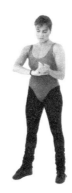

USE THE SECOND HAND OF A WATCH OR CLOCK TO CHECK YOUR PULSE. If you are above the upper limit of your exercise training zone, slow the pace and tone down the moves. If you are below the lower limit of your range, step up your movements and exaggerate your arm motions.

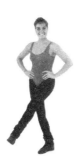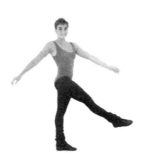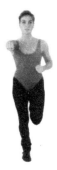

15. Hands on hips, kick out lightly to the right and then to the left, 4 times each.

16. Continue the light kicking motion, adding arms swinging high overhead, alternating to right and left sides, 12 times each side; then swing your arms overhead and down 16 times.

17. Keep moving your feet and punch out to the left 4 times and then the right 4 times.

18. With arms swinging, take 3 quick steps forward to the right and kick; then take 3 quick steps to the left, kick and reverse. Repeat 8 times in each direction.

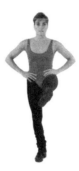

19. Bring your feet together and jog in time to the music. Then step sideways, take quick steps right, left, and right again and high kick forward, quick-step left, right, left, and high-kick forward again in time to the beat. Do 8 kicks with each foot; then repeat the step and kick sideways, 8 times each side.

20. Run forward 4 steps, kick forward, then back 4 steps and kick forward again, swinging your arms up and down as you move.

21. Standing in place, lift your knees to your chest alternately, arms swinging down as each knee comes up.

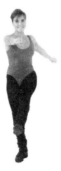
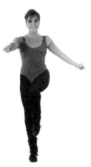

22. Do quick toe-heel jog-steps in place, first swinging your arms lightly for 16 counts and then swinging them high overhead and down 16 times.

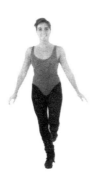 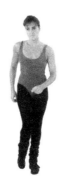

23. Kick your heels backward, alternating your feet, arms moving up and down to the side.

24. Lift your left knee and then kick left. Then repeat to the right, 8 times for each side.

TAKE PULSE COUNT.

25. Keep your feet moving in place and move into a toe-heel jogging step. Move 3 steps to the right and kick; then move 3 to the left and kick. Repeat 12 times in each direction.

26. Skip in place 8 times; then skip 4 steps forward and 4 steps back. Skip in place again, swinging your arms overhead and down. Then repeat the 1-2-3 kick steps to right and left, 8 more times to each side. As you kick, punch out with your arms.

27. Jog in place and do double bounces in place, with your arms alternately swinging up and down for 30 seconds.

28. Punch right and then left. Repeat 8 times for each side.

29. Jog in place, moving your arms up and down in front of you and then up and down to the sides.

30. Kick to the beat, alternating your legs and punching out with your arms to the left and then to the right for 8 kicks. Follow by swinging your arms up and down for 8 more kicks.

31. Jog lightly for several circles around the room; then slow to a walk.

Unless otherwise noted, each step should be repeated 8 times in each direction. (End with slower music.)

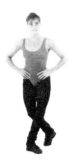 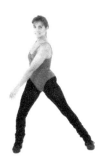

1. Step to the left and then to the right, swinging your arms.

2. March easily, 4 steps forward, 4 steps back.

3. Do a sideways chain step (one foot in front of the other and then one foot back).

4. Stand with your legs apart and lunge from side to side slowly swinging your arms.

5. Bend your knees while lifting and lowering your arms.

6. Place your hands against a wall or hold on to a chair back to stretch your calves. Lean away and lift and press alternate heels down; then press down both heels.

7. With your back to a wall or your hands on the back of a chair, lean on your heels to stretch your toes.

8. Pull in your right knee and hold it against your chest. Repeat with your left knee.

9. Stand with your feet apart and reach for the ceiling, inhaling as you reach up and exhaling as you bring your arms down. Repeat 3 times.

CHECK PULSE. If it is not below 20, continue walking around the room for a minute longer and then check it again.

CONTROLLED-IMPACT AEROBICS

Controlled-impact aerobics are equally valuable aerobic workouts with similar movements done to music, but the movements are modified to eliminate jogging, jumping, and other movements that jar the body. Instead, one foot always remains firmly on the floor and the arms work harder. Following are some suggested controlled-impact steps that you can work into a home dance routine. You will see that many steps are similar to regular aerobics, but adapted to eliminate jarring. Repeat each routine 8 times.

Controlled-Impact Aerobic Workout

STEP TOUCH

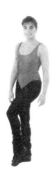 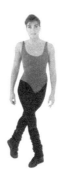

1. Step sideways right and bring your left toe to your right foot; reverse to the left. Vary by stepping and pointing toes in front of the body and in back of the body, stepping and reaching heels in front of the body.

2. Add arms forward, up and open to the side, one at a time and then both together.

3. Swing one or both arms from side to side.

STEP KICK

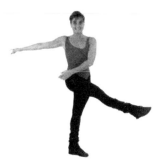

1. Kick forward, alternating your legs. With kicks, alternately push your arms forward either at diagonals, straight out, to the sides, or up in the air.

MARCH/WALK

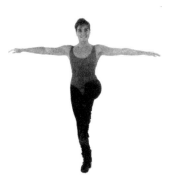 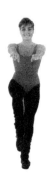 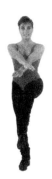

1. While briskly marching in place, do the following arm movements:
Move your arms up, out to the side, down, and then out to the side.
Scissor your arms forward.
Pull your elbows back and then extend your arms.

2. March forward 4 steps and back 4 steps, scissoring up as you go forward and down as you move backward.

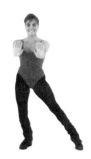

3. Step forward 3 steps; then lift one knee. Take 3 steps back and repeat the knee lift. Alternate legs.

4. Again step forward 3 steps and kick on the fourth beat. Take 3 steps back and repeat the kick. Alternate legs.

5. Walk forward 4 steps and touch each leg out to the side. Walk back 4 steps and repeat the side touches, adding arm presses with each touch. (To do an arm press, extend your arms to the side at shoulder level and flex at the elbow so your fingers point toward the ceiling. Keeping your upper arms at shoulder height, bring your lower arms together in front of your face until your elbows meet. Return to the starting position.)

6. Repeat any of these routines moving 4 steps to each side instead of back and forth.

KNEE LIFTS

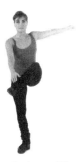

1. Lift each knee alternately and then lift each knee 2 times.

2. Touch your ankles with each lift.

3. Lift your arms high above your head and pull down with each knee lift.

4. Let your arms swing from side to side with the lifts.

SKI POLE

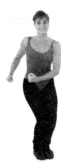

1. Keeping your feet together, reach your arms over your head and pull down to the sides.

2. Using a ski pole motion, plant your arm down, kicking your other leg out to the side. Twist and repeat to the other side.

TOUCH STEP

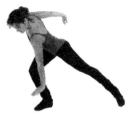

1. Reach your foot out to the side of your body; then step in place, alternating sides.

2. Add arm movements, swinging your arms diagonally across your body, above your head, or reaching down toward the floor.

3. Take 3 steps right and touch-step. Repeat to the left, with your arms reaching in the same direction as the steps.

STEP KICK-UP

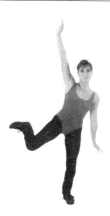

1. Step out to one side and kick opposite leg up toward your buttocks.

2. Add arm swings down in front of your body and then up, to the side, and overhead.

ROCK STEP

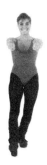 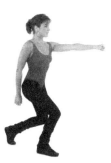

1. Place your weight on your right foot; then rock back and place your weight on your left foot.

2. Add punching motions with one and then both arms.

CHARLESTON STEP

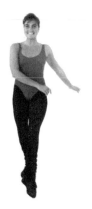 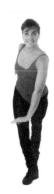

1. Step right, point forward to the left; step left and point back to the right.

2. Step forward with one leg and then back on the same leg, with arms swinging in the direction of each move.

3. Do 3 march steps forward and then the Charleston step. Repeat marching back.

4. Do complete arm circles with each front rock step.

HIP ROCKS

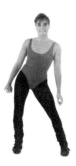 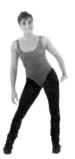

1. Swing your hips from side to side, keeping the top half of your body still.

2. Add arm movements up and then down as though dribbling a basketball.

CALISTHENICS

Calisthenics are exercises that improve fitness levels by increasing strength and muscular endurance. They also tone and firm the muscles. If you continue a regular program of calisthenics, you will see changes in your body even if you do not lose weight. Your figure will be trimmer, and your clothes will fit better as lumps and bumps start to disappear.

At Palm-Aire, exercise workouts are keyed to the fitness level of each guest. "Spa I" is for beginners, "Spa II" is for the basic intermediate workout for all the major muscle groups, and "Spa III" is an advanced set of exercises that increases the intensity of the workout even more by adding the resistance of free weights to strengthen and firm muscles.

At every level, each set of exercises works specific muscles. The key to getting the best results is to learn to perform the exercises with what is known as "dynamic tension." This means maintaining the muscle's tension through the entire range of motions. To accomplish this, do each exercise in a slow, controlled manner, keeping the muscles tense, rather than working faster with less control, which allows momentum to do part of the work.

Each exercise should be repeated 8 to 16 times. As you get stronger, you will be able to maintain a greater degree of tension in the muscle, making the workout more and more effective without adding repetitions.

Palm-Aire instructors never urge exercisers to "go for the burn," which means continuing to exercise until it hurts. You need not hurt for an exercise to be beneficial. It is far more important to build up your capacity slowly. To do this, at each workout try for just 1 or 2 more repetitions than you did comfortably at the previous workout. This is what is often called the *training effect*. By stretching your capacity just a little more each session, you will gradually increase the muscle's capacity. Once the first few days pass, you will see that you will be able to do more repetitions comfortably with each passing day.

To avoid injuries and get maximum benefits, it is important that each exercise is done in the proper position, as illustrated on the following page:

BASIC EXERCISE POSITIONS

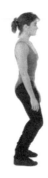

STANDING PELVIC TILT POSITION

BACK-LYING POSITIONS

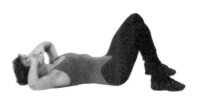

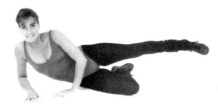

SIDE-LYING POSITION

ALL FOURS POSITION

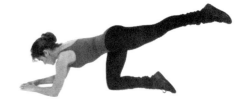

The following exercises are for strengthening and firming your muscles. The wand is used to ensure correct body alignment and positioning. The exercises should be performed in a controlled manner, concentrating on the muscles being utilized. Repeat each exercise 8 to 16 times.

SHOULDERS, CHEST, ARMS, AND UPPER BACK

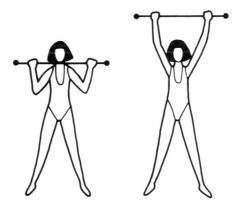

• *Overhead press.* With the wand parallel to the floor, hands slightly more than shoulder distance apart, and palms facing the floor, raise and lower the wand from chest level to a straight-arm position overhead. Return to the starting position.

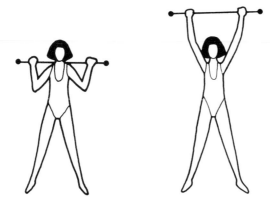

- *Variation*. Bring the wand down behind your neck and then press up.

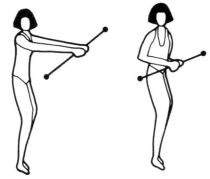

- *Chest press*. With the wand parallel to the floor, and your hands slightly more than shoulder distance apart, palms facing the floor, press the wand straight out in front of your body; then return to the starting position.

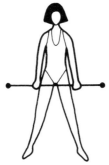

- *Straight arm lift*. With your hands on the wand approximately shoulder distance apart, extend your arms toward the floor; keeping arms straight, raise the wand overhead. Return to the starting position.

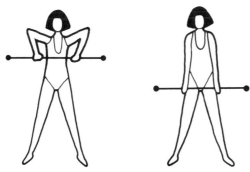

• *Tricep push*. With your hands in the center of the wand, raise the wand to chin level, your elbows lifted higher than the wand; then with a pressing motion, push the wand toward the floor. Return to the starting position.

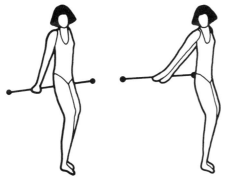

• *Tricep lift*. With the wand placed behind your body, palms facing the ceiling, hands approximately shoulder distance apart, lift the wand away from your body. Return to the starting position.

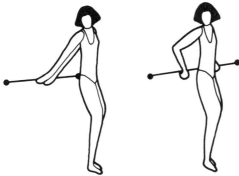

• *Tricep extension*. With the wand placed behind your body, palms facing the ceiling, hands approximately shoulder distance apart, lift the wand by bending your elbows; then extend your arms down. Return to the starting position.

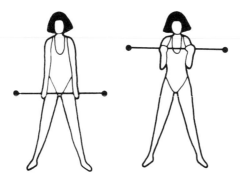

- *Bicep Curl*. With your hands on the wand about shoulder distance apart, palms facing up, keep your upper arms next to your sides, and lift the wand to your shoulders. Return to the starting position.

HIPS, THIGHS, AND BUTTOCKS

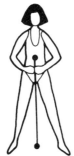 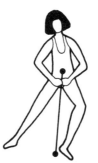 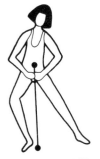

- *Lunges*. Place the wand in front of you perpendicular to the floor. With hands resting lightly on top, legs in a comfortable wide-stride position, bend your right knee, distributing the body weight to the right leg. Your body should remain vertical and your knee should bend directly over the right foot. Return to the starting position and repeat to the left side.

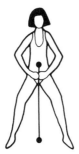

- *Plies*. Place the wand in front of your body, perpendicular to the floor, with your hands resting lightly on top, legs in a comfortable stride position. Lower your hips by bending your knees—keep your heels on the floor—squeeze your buttocks together. Return to the starting position.

THIGHS

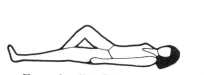 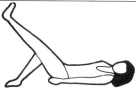

• *Front leg lift.* Lie on your back with your right leg bent, the foot flat on the floor, and your left leg extended. Slowly lift and lower your extended leg. Return to the starting position and repeat on the other side.

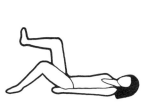 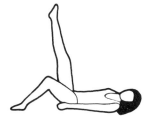

• *Leg extensions.* Lie on your back with your right leg bent and the foot flat on the floor. Your left leg should be in the table-top position. Extend your left leg toward the ceiling. Return to the starting position. Alternate legs.

INNER THIGHS

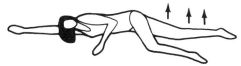

• *Inner thigh lift.* Lie on your side and cross your top leg over your bottom leg in front of your body. Lift and lower bottom leg, trying not to rest leg on floor as your lower it. Roll to your other side and repeat the exercise with your other leg.

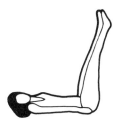 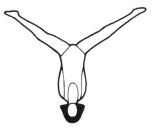

• *Inner thigh straddles.* Lie on your back with legs perpendicular to the floor, knees slightly bent. Open and close your legs in scissor fashion. Keep your lower back pressed to the floor and abdominals contracted.

61

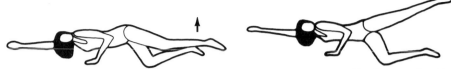

• *Side leg lifts*. Lie on your side with your hips perpendicular to the floor. Rest your head on your arm and bend your bottom leg to help maintain balance. Lift and lower the top leg in a slow, controlled manner. Roll to your other side and repeat exercise with your other leg.

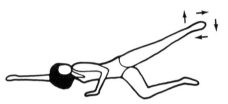

• *Variations*. Lift your leg up and draw squares with your lifted leg. Lift your leg and do small lifts with the elevated leg.

BUTTOCKS

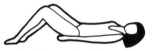 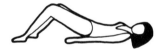

• *Pelvic tucks*. Lie on your back with your knees bent and feet flat on the floor. Press your navel toward your spine and at the same time contract your buttock muscles slightly off the ground, hold and release. (*Note:* The lower back should always remain in contact with the floor.)

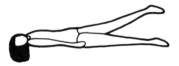

• *Back leg lifts*. Lie face down on the floor (head remains down) and place a pillow, towels, or hands under your abdominals. Pressing hips toward the floor, contract your buttock muscles, causing your leg to lift slightly off the floor. Repeat with your other leg.

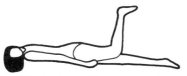

• *Variation*. Flex your leg at the knee and press your foot toward the ceiling.

ABDOMINALS

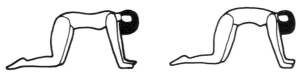

ISOMETRIC CONTRACTIONS

• *Cat arch*. Assume the all-fours position, with back flat and head aligned with back. Contract abdominal muscles, pulling back up and rounding shoulders like an angry cat. Hold for a count of 8, while continuing to breathe normally. Release and repeat 4 to 8 times.

• *Pelvic tilt*. Lie on your back with your knees bent and your feet flat on the floor. Contract abdominals, pressing the small of your back firmly to the floor. Hold for a count of 8, while continuing to breathe normally. Release and repeat 4 to 8 times.

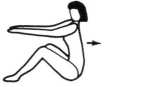
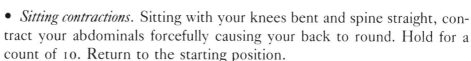

• *Sitting contractions*. Sitting with your knees bent and spine straight, contract your abdominals forcefully causing your back to round. Hold for a count of 10. Return to the starting position.

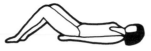 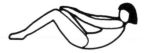

CURL-UP

• *Level* 1. Lie on your back with your knees bent and your feet flat on the floor. Place your hands on your thighs and gently lift your head and shoulders off the floor, reaching your hands toward your knees. Hold for a count of 10. Return to the starting position.

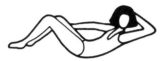

• *Level* 2. This is the same as level 1, except that one arm is extended and the other supports your head by placing the hand behind the neck cradling your head in your arm. Breathe normally as you reach your extended arm forward and lift your head and shoulders. Return to the starting position and repeat for your other arm.

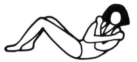

• *Level* 3. This is the same as level 1, except that your arms are crossed over your chest. Lift and lower your head and shoulders off the floor continuing to breathe normally.

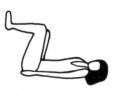 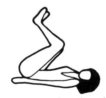

• *Reverse curl-ups.* Lie on your back with your knees bent into your chest, arms beside your hips, palms down. Lift your hips off the floor and slowly return to the starting position.

Spa II—Intermediate-Level Exercises

The following exercises are for strengthening and firming your muscles. We suggest that you perform these exercises with what is known as "dynamic tension." This means that the muscles' ability to maintain tension throughout the entire range of motion is utilized. The exercises should be performed in a slow, controlled manner with the muscles tensed the entire time (working faster and with less control usually allows momentum—not you—to do part of the work). Repeat each exercise 8 to 16 times. As you get stronger, you will be able to maintain a greater degree of tension in the muscle, thus continuing to make your workout effective without adding repetitions.

SHOULDERS, CHEST, ARMS, AND UPPER BACK

(All upper body work should be done with shoulders relaxed, knees slightly bent, and abdominals contracted.)

ARMS

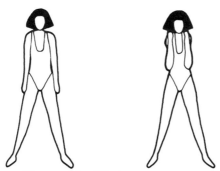

• *Bicep curls.* With your upper arms held firmly next to your sides, flex and extend your lower arms. Return to the starting position.

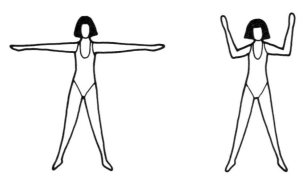

• *Variation.* Extend your arms out to the side and flex and extend your lower arm, keeping your upper arms still.

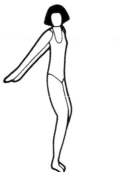

• *Tricep extension*. Extend your arms straight behind your body. With your upper arms remaining still, flex and extend your lower arms. Return to the starting position.

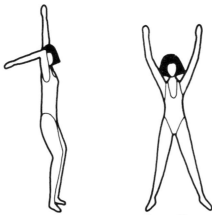

• *Overhead tricep extensions*. Extend your arms straight overhead. Keeping your upper arms still, bend your elbow as if to pat yourself on the back; then extend your arm straight overhead. Return to the starting position and repeat exercise with your other arm.

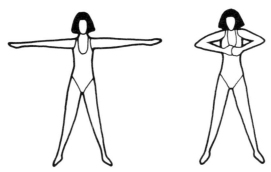

• *Lateral tricep extensions*. With your arms extended out to the sides, keep your upper arms still and pull your lower arms toward your body; then return to starting position.

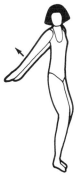

• *Tricep lifts*. Extend your arms straight behind your body. Lift and lower your arms with controlled movements, maintaining the tension in your muscles. Return to the starting position.

SHOULDERS AND UPPER BACK

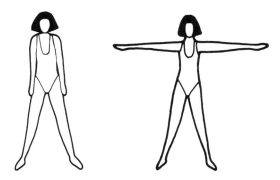

• *Lateral arm raises*. Start with your arms down by your sides. Lift your straight arms out to side at shoulder height. Return to the starting position.

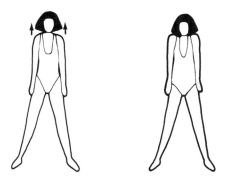

• *Shoulder raises*. Lift your shoulders toward your ears and return to the starting position.

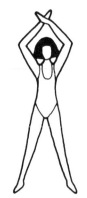 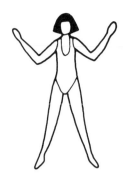

• *Pull-downs*. Starting with your arms overhead and hands crossed, pull your arms down by flexing your elbows and squeezing your shoulder blades together. Return to the starting position.

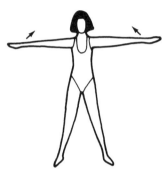

• *Shoulder-blade squeeze*. Extend your arms out to the side parallel to ground, palms facing back. Squeeze your shoulder blades together. Return to the position.

CHEST

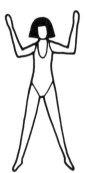 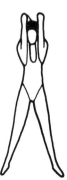

• *Chest press*. Extend your arms to the side at shoulder level and flex at the elbow so your fingers point toward the ceiling. Keeping your upper arms at shoulder height, bring your lower arms together in front of your face. Return to the starting position.

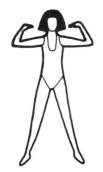 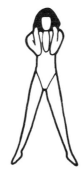

- *Chest crossover.* Put your hands on your shoulders, elbows pressed out to either side at shoulder height. Bring your elbows together in front of your chest, crossing your elbows alternately right over left and then left over right.

HIPS, THIGHS, AND BUTTOCKS

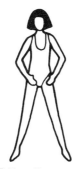 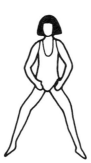

- *Plies.* Separate your legs in a comfortable straddle position. Lower your hips by bending your knees. Keep your heels on the floor and your knees extended directly over your feet. Return to the starting position.

THIGHS

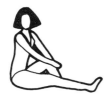

- *Sitting quadracep lift.* Sit on the floor with your right leg bent and your foot flat on the floor, arms hugging your leg, and your left leg extended. Lift and lower your extended leg. Repeat for the other side.

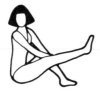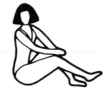

• *Sitting quadracep presses.* Sit on the floor with your right leg bent and your foot flat on the floor, arms hugging your leg, and your left leg extended. Lift extended leg; then flex leg and pull it in toward your body, return to straight leg lifted position. Repeat for other leg.

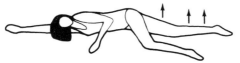

• *Inner thigh lifts.* Lie on your side and cross your top leg over your bottom leg in front of your body. Flex your bottom leg slightly and lift and lower it with controlled motions. Roll over and repeat the exercise with your other leg.

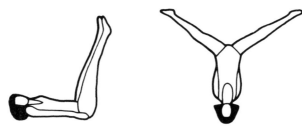

• *Inner thigh straddles.* Lie on your back with your legs perpendicular to the floor and your knees slightly bent. Open and close your legs in scissor fashion, keeping your lower back pressed to the floor and abdominals contracted.

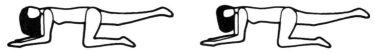

• *Hamstring pulls.* Assume a modified all-fours position (weight on knees and forearms) and extend one leg behind your body at hip level. Keeping your knee level with your hip, bring your heel toward your buttocks. Return to the starting position. Repeat the exercise with your other leg.

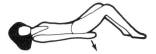

- *Pelvic tucks.* Lie on your back with your knees bent and your feet flat on the floor. Press your navel toward your spine and, at the same time, contract your buttock muscles lifting slightly off the floor; hold and release. (*Note:* the lower back always remains in contact with the floor.)

Variation a   *Variation b*

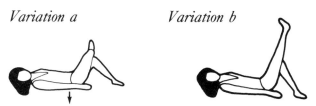

- *Variations.* (a) Cross one leg over the other, continue to contract and release. (b) Extend one leg straight into the air and continue to contract and release.

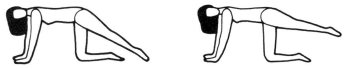

- *Back leg lifts.* Assume the all-fours position, weight evenly distributed, and extend one leg behind your body, toe resting on the floor. Lift your leg to hip level by contracting your buttock muscles; then lower in a slow controlled manner. Repeat the exercise with your other leg.

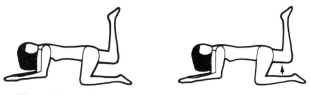

- *Footprints.* Assume a modified all-fours position (weight on knees and forearms), extend one leg behind your body at hip level, flex at the knee so your foot is toward the ceiling, contract your buttocks, causing the foot to be lifted slightly toward the ceiling. Repeat the exercise with your other leg.

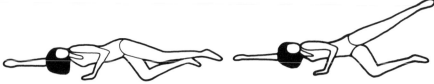

- *Side leg lifts.* Lie on your side with your hips perpendicular to the floor, head resting on an arm, and bottom leg bent to help maintain balance. Lift and lower your top leg with slow, controlled movements. Roll to your other side and repeat the exercise with your other leg.

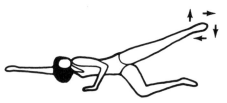

- *Variation.* Lift your leg up and draw a square with your lifted leg; hold for 10 seconds, or do small lifts.

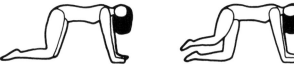

- *Side fire-hydrants.* Assume the all-fours position, weight evenly distributed, and lift flexed leg to side and lower without resting on the floor. Return to the starting position and repeat exercise with your other leg.

ABDOMINALS

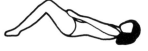 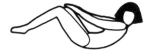

CURL-UP/CRUNCH.
- *Level* 1. Lie on your back with your knees bent and your feet flat on the floor. Place your hands on your thighs and gently lift your head and shoulders off the floor, reaching your hands toward your knees. Hold, then return to the starting position.

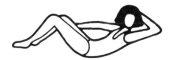

- *Level* 2. Same as level 1, except one arm is extended and the other is placed behind your neck. Reach your extended arm forward as you lift your head and shoulders.

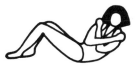

- *Level* 3. Same as level 1, except your arms are crossed over your chest. Lift and lower your head and shoulders off the floor.

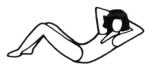

- *Level* 4. Same as level 1, except both of your arms are above your head, fingertips on your temples.

Variation a   *Variation b*   *Variation c*

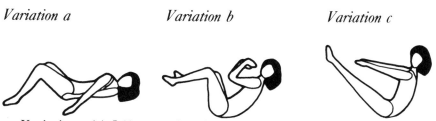

- *Variations.* (a) Lift your head and one shoulder off the floor, reaching your arm across your body. (b) Legs in table-top position, curlup and touch your elbow to your knees. (c) Extend your legs straight up into the air with a slight bend in the knee and reach for your ankles.

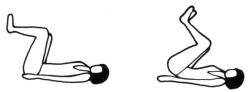

- *Reverse curl-up/crunch.* Lie on your back with your knees bent into your chest. Place your hands palms-down on the floor and lift your hips off the floor and then slowly return to the starting position.

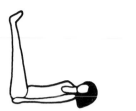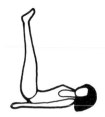

• *Variation*. Extend your legs toward the ceiling. Lifting your hips off the floor, reach your feet toward the ceiling, not diagonally toward your head. Return to the starting position.

SHIN STRENGTHENERS
(These aid in the prevention of shin injuries.)

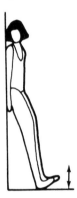

• *Wall lean*. Leaning on the wall, with your feet about 2 feet in front of your body, lift your toes up and down (both at the same time).

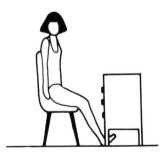

• *Isometric lift*. Place your toes under an immovable object, such as a sofa, or desk. Press your toes as if you are trying to lift the immovable source.

Spa III—Advanced-Level Exercises

The following exercises use the added resistance of free weights to strengthen and firm muscles. For effectiveness and safety it is essential that proper body alignment is maintained. Only the muscles involved in the exercise are used; the rest of the body remains still. All exercises should be performed in a slow, controlled manner. Start with 3-pound hand weights and 2½-pound leg weights. Each exercise should be repeated 8 to 16 times. When this has been mastered with good form, heavier weights may be used if further strength gains are desired.

SHOULDERS, CHEST, ARMS, AND UPPER BACK

(All upper body work should be done with shoulders relaxed, knees slightly bent, and abdominals contracted.)

ARMS

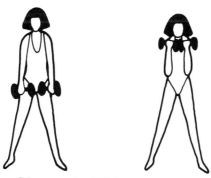

• *Bicep curls*. With your upper arms held firmly next to your sides, flex and extend your lower arms. Return to starting position.

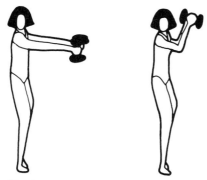

• *Variation*. Extend your arms out in front of you and flex and extend your lower arms, keeping your upper arms still.

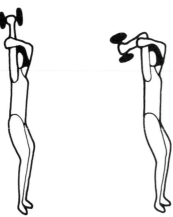

• *Overhead tricep extensions.* Hold the weight in one hand and extend your arm straight overhead. Stabilizing your elbow with your opposite hand, lower the weight behind your back; then extend it above your head. Return to the starting position and repeat the exercise with your other arm.

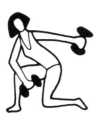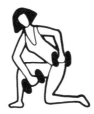

• *Tricep extensions.* Kneel on the floor on one leg with your other leg bent with the foot flat on the floor. Leaning on your bent leg with one arm, extend the other arm with the weight straight behind your body. Keep your upper arm still and flex and extend your elbow, moving only your lower arm. Return to the starting position and repeat the exercise with your other arm.

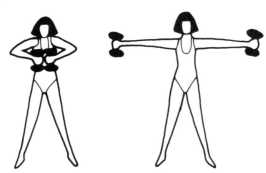

• *Lateral tricep extension.* With your arms extended out to your sides, keep your upper arms still and pull your lower arms toward your body at chest level. Return to the starting position.

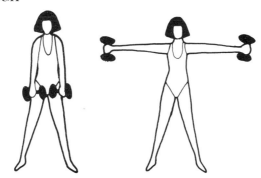

• *Lateral arm raises*. Start with your arms down by your sides. Lift your arms straight away from your sides to shoulder height and lower your arms back down to your sides.

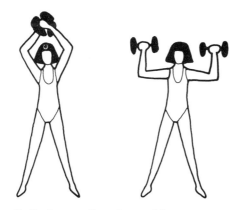

• *Pull-downs*. Starting with your arms overhead and your hands crossed, pull your arms down by flexing your elbows and squeezing your shoulder blades together. Return to the starting position.

CHEST

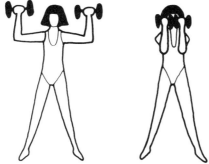

• *Chest press*. With your arms extended out to the side, elbows flexed so fingers point toward the ceiling, and keeping your upper arms at shoulder height, bring your lower arms together in front of your face. Return to the starting position.

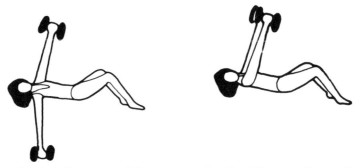

• *Supine chest press.* Lie on your back with your knees bent and your feet flat on the floor, arms out to the side at shoulder height. With a slight bend in your elbows, lift the weights toward the ceiling. Return to the starting position. This exercise is especially effective when performed slowly.

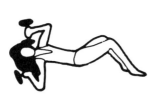
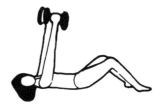

• *Bench press.* Lying on your back with your elbows bent and your hands near your shoulders, press the weights straight toward the ceiling. Return to the starting position.

ABDOMINALS

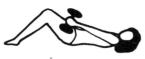
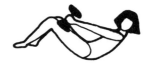

CURL-UP/CRUNCH.

• *Basic crunch.* Lie on your back with your knees bent, your feet flat on the floor, and weights in your hands. Place your hands on either side of your legs and gently lift your head and shoulders off the floor, reaching your hands past your knees. Hold for a count of 10. Return to the starting position.

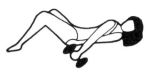 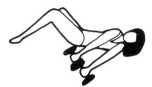 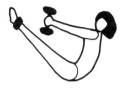

• *Variations*. (a) Same as basic crunch, except only one shoulder lifts off the floor, reaching your arm across your body. (b) Same as basic crunch, except one or both arms reach to the opposite side of your body. (c) Extend your legs straight up into the air with a slight bend in your knees (hand and leg weights optional).

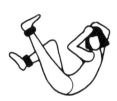 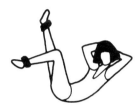

• *Bicycles*. Lie on your back with one leg bent into your chest and one extended toward the ceiling (leg weights on both ankles, no hand weights). With head and shoulders lifted off the floor (fingertips on temples), alternately straighten and bend your legs, touching your opposite elbow to your knee.

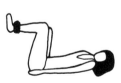

• *Reverse curl-up*. Lie on your back with your knees bent into your chest, leg weights on both ankles. Place your hands palm-down next to your sides and lift your hips off the floor, drawing your knees toward your chest. Slowly return to the starting position.

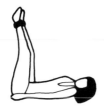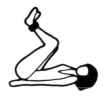

• *Variation*. Extend your legs toward the ceiling. Lifting your hips off the floor, reach your feet toward the ceiling.

HIPS, THIGHS, AND BUTTOCKS

(All of the following exercises are performed with weights securely fastened around your ankles.)

THIGHS

• *Sitting quadracep lifts*. Sit on the floor with your left leg bent, foot flat on the floor, arms hugging your leg, and your opposite leg extended in front of your body with a slight bend in the knee. Lift and lower your extended leg. Repeat the exercise with your other leg.

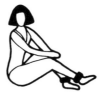

• *Sitting quadracep presses*. Sit on the floor with your left leg bent, foot flat on the floor, arms hugging your leg, and your opposite leg extended in front of your body with a slight bend in the knee. Flex your leg and pull your extended leg in toward your body. Return to the starting position. Repeat the exercise with your other leg.

INNER THIGHS

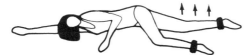

- *Inner thigh lifts*. Lie on your side and cross your top leg over your bottom leg in front of your body. Flex your bottom leg slightly and lift and lower it with controlled motions. Roll to your other side and repeat the exercise with your other leg.

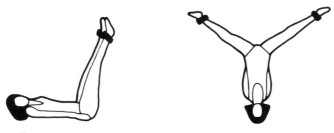

- *Inner thigh straddles*. Lie on your back with legs perpendicular to the floor, knees slightly bent. Open and close your legs in scissor fashion. Keep your lower back pressed to the floor and abdominals contracted.

BUTTOCKS AND HAMSTRINGS

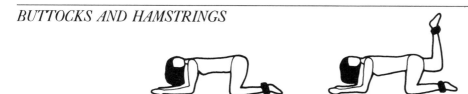

- *Back leg lifts*. Modified all-fours position, weight evenly distributed, and keeping leg flexed, lift your knee to buttocks level. Return to starting position. Repeat the exercise with your other leg.

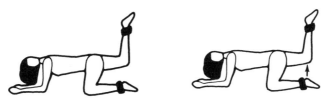

- *Footprints*. In a modified all-fours position (weight on knees and forearms), extend one leg behind your body at hip level, flex your knee so the bottom of your foot is toward the ceiling. Contract buttocks, causing foot to be lifted slightly toward the ceiling. Repeat the exercise with your other leg.

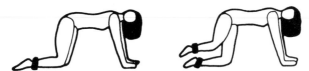

• *Side fire-hydrants*. Assume the all-fours position, weight evenly distributed, and lift flexed leg to side and lower without resting leg on floor. Return to the starting position and repeat the exercise with your other leg.

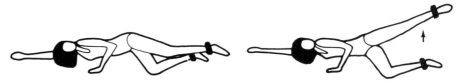

• *Side leg lifts*. Lie on your side, hips perpendicular to the floor, head resting on your arm, and bottom leg bent to help maintain balance. Lift and lower top leg slowly controlling the movement. Roll to your other side and repeat the exercise with your other leg.

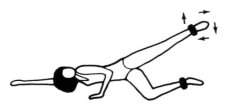

• *Variations*. Lift your leg up and draw squares, hold, or do small lifts.

WATER EXERCISES

Water is an excellent medium for both strength/firming type exercises and for aerobic exercise. The effort you use to pull your body through the water will determine the resistance created by the water. Therefore, many fitness levels can be accommodated in one class. The water also offers effective cushioning for sensitive joint areas and dissipates body heat for a cool comfortable workout.

The starred (*) exercises may also be appropriate for water aerobic activities.

Free-Standing Exercises

All of the following arm exercises should be performed with abdominals tight, buttocks tucked, feet shoulder width or more apart, knees bent, and shoulders under the water. Repeat each exercise 8 times.

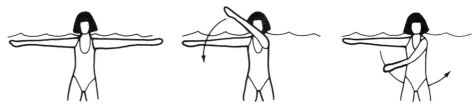

ARM SWEEPS   With your arms at shoulder height out to the side, stretch your right arm overhead to your left arm and sweep your right arm (palm first) through the water to the right. Repeat with left arm.

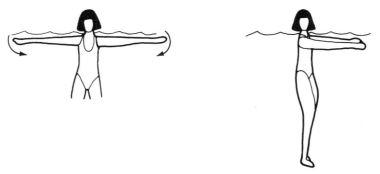

WATER PULL   With your arms out to the side at shoulder height, cup your hands and pull water forward; then turn your palms away and pull water backward.

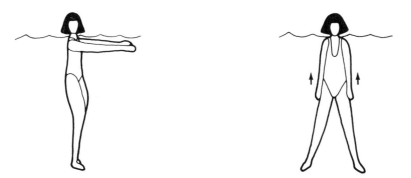

SKI PULL   With your arms out to the front and palms down, pull your arms down to your sides; then turn your palms up, pulling your arms to the surface.

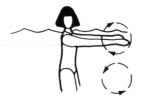 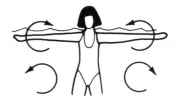 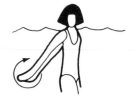

ARM CIRCLES   a. Extend your arms in front of your body, palms toward the bottom of the pool, and circle your arms inward and then outward.

b. Extend your arms to the side, palms toward the bottom of the pool, and circle your arms forward and backward.

c. Extend your arms behind your body, palms up, and circle your arms inward and then outward.

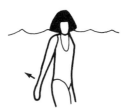 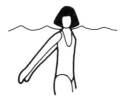

TRICEP PUSHES   With your arms down by your sides, palms facing back, press your arms further back. Return to starting position.

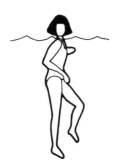

*JOG   Jog around the pool, keeping abdominals contracted.

- *Variations:* a. Jog backward.
  - b. Jog with arms overhead.
  - c. Jog with the following arms strokes: front crawl, breast stroke, butterfly, backstroke.

84

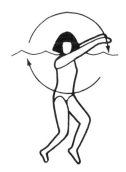

JUMP WAVES   Leap forward in the water and simultaneously pull the water back with a front crawl, butterfly, or breaststroke.

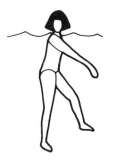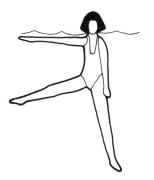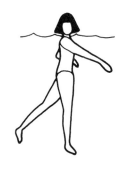

LEG KICKS   Hop and kick legs.
- a. Kick front and reach with opposite arm.
- b. Kick side and reach with same arm.
- c. Kick back and push opposite arm to the front.

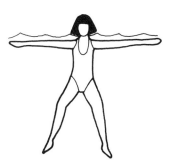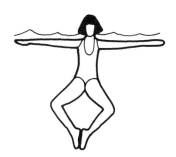

FROG   With your feet in a comfortable wide-stride position and your arms extended out to the sides, lift your feet, bringing the soles of your feet together; then extend your legs to the starting position.

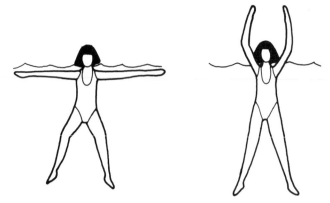

JUMPING JACKS   With your feet shoulder width apart and your arms at shoulder height, bring your feet together and at the same time extend your arms overhead and clap.

- *Variations.* a. Bring your feet together and pull your arms down to meet under the water.

  b. As your feet come together, cross your right foot in front of your left and then alternate.

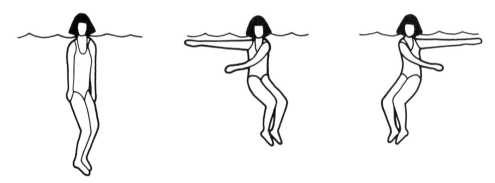

WAIST TWISTER   Keeping your feet together, with knees slightly bent, twist side to side, while pulling your arms in the opposite direction.

Bar Exercises

All bar exercises should be done with correct posture: shoulders relaxed, abdominals contracted, and buttocks tucked under.

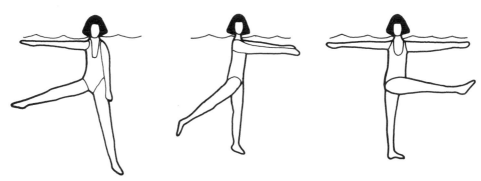

LEG LIFTS With your toe pointed, lift your leg toward the surface of the water—front, back, or side.

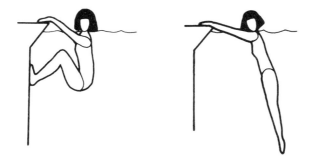

KNEES TO CHEST With your feet on the wall, roll out, touching your feet to the bottom of the pool behind you; then pull back in with tight abdominals.

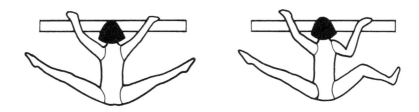

LUNGES ON WALL With your feet on the wall and with a wide straddle position (shoulders under the water), bend your right leg while keeping your left leg straight and move to the right. Repeat to the left.

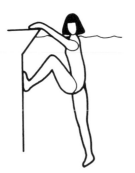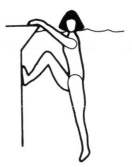

*MOUNTAIN
CLIMBER

With your left foot on the bottom of the pool and your right foot on the wall, jump and change leg positions.

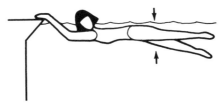

*FLUTTER
KICKS

Hold on to the bar and extend your feet behind you. Kick your feet in a flutter motion.

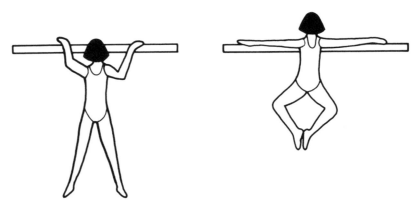

*JUMP-UP
FROG KICKS

Face the bar and hold it with both hands. Propel your body up and out of the pool by jumping and bringing your feet toward your buttocks, keeping your knees out to the side.

88

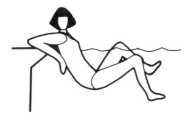

*BICYCLE   Turn so that your back is to the bar. Lower your elbows to the bar and support your weight on the bar. Pull your knees to your chest and move your legs in a bicycling motion.

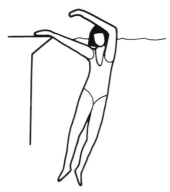

SIDE STRETCHES With your feet together and close to the wall, hold the bar with your left hand. Lean your hips away from the bar and stretch your right arm over your right ear toward the bar. Repeat for the other side.

Ball Exercises

When performing the following exercises, your knees should be bent, abdominals tight, and shoulders relaxed.

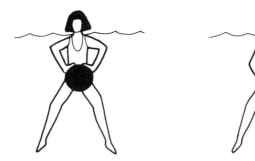

TRICEP PUSH   Place your hands on top of the ball with your fingers pointing toward the center (elbows pressed to sides). Push the ball below your hip level and allow it slowly to come back to just below the surface.

89

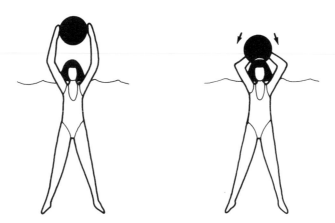

TRICEP
EXTENSION

With both arms overhead, and your hands on either side of the ball, lower the ball behind your head and lift it. Be sure to keep your elbows as close to your head as possible. Return to the starting position and repeat.

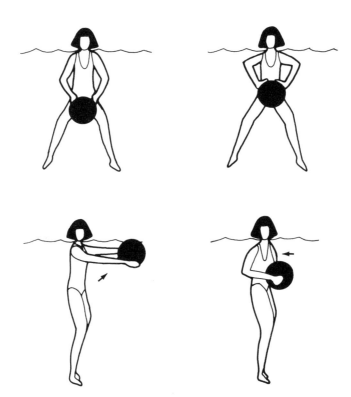

PECTORAL PUSH Place your hands on the sides of the ball with your elbows up. Push the ball downward to just below your navel, then straight out, upward, and then inward to your chest. Return to the starting position and repeat.

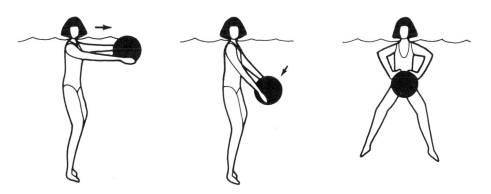

ALTERNATE
PECTORAL PUSH   Reverse the motion of the above exercise, moving the ball out, down, and then in.

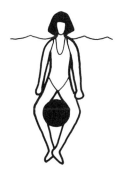

"CHARLIE
CHAPLIN"   Place the ball between your knees and press inward. Keep your heels together, toes pointed, and walk flat-footed around the pool.

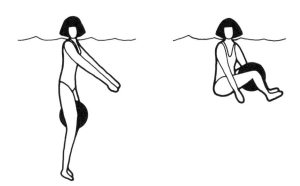

• *Variation.* Take the same initial position as above and then pull your knees to your chest and lower them.

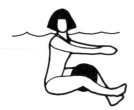

*SITTING
BREAST STROKE

In a sitting position, hold the ball tightly with your legs. Cross your ankles, allowing your feet to float up, and do a breaststroke with your arms,
for 10 to 15 seconds.

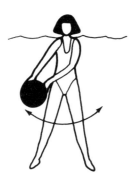

"AROUND
THE WORLD"

With your hands on the sides of the ball and feet shoulder-width apart,
extend your arms to the sides and move the ball from left to right.

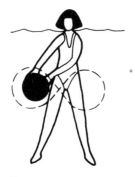

FIGURE 8

Place the ball under the water and make a figure 8 from side to side.

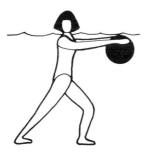

*LEAP   Reach forward, holding the ball in both hands, and push the ball under the water, while leaping forward.

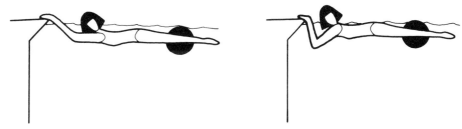

PULL-UPS   Face the bar. With the ball held firmly between your knees, allow your hips and feet to float behind you. Extend your arms and pull your body into the bar; then push away from the bar with your arms.

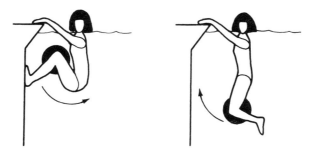

ABDOMINAL TUCKS   Face the bar. With the ball held firmly between your knees, pull your knees to your chest and bring your feet to the wall. Push off, just so your knees point toward the bottom of the pool; then bring your legs back to the starting position.

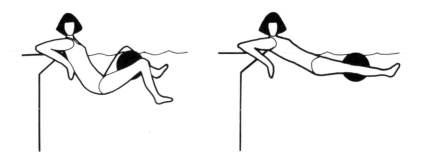

KNEE TUCKS　　Place the ball between your knees and cross your ankles. Put your back to the bar and extend your arms comfortably along the bar. Pull your knees into your chest, tightening the abdominals; then extend your legs to the starting position.

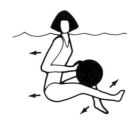

***HUGS**　　Hold the ball close to your chest, extend your legs out to the front, and kick vigorously, propelling yourself backward.

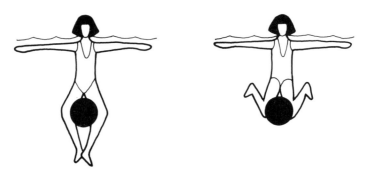

HAMSTRING TUCKS　　With the ball between knees, bring your heels up toward your buttocks. With your arms out for balance, lower your feet and repeat.

94

Kickboard Exercises

For most of the following exercises, two Styrofoam kickboards are required. A kickboard is placed under each arm so that the body is supported on both the upper arm and the forearm. Both arms and shoulders should remain relaxed as the lower body is exercised. The proper arm position is illustrated below.

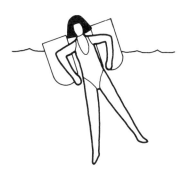

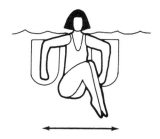

KNEES TO
CHEST TWIST   With your knees tucked into your chest, twist your body from side to side. Remember to pull the abdominal muscles in tightly.

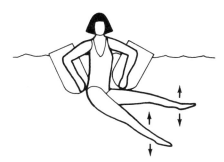

*FLUTTER KICK   Sitting up (your body should look like an **L**), flutter kick from the hip, using your entire leg. Repeat the exercise with your other leg.

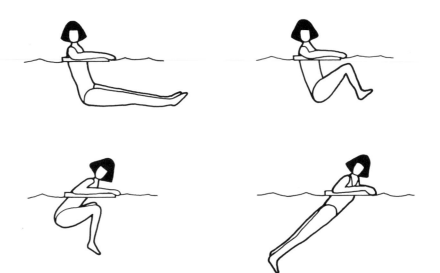

ROCKING CHAIR   With your legs together and in front of your body, bend your knees to your chest and lean your body weight forward; then extend your legs toward the back and down toward the bottom of the pool. Repeat 8 times.

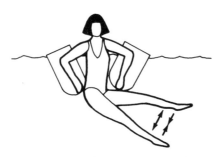

STRADDLE
PULLS   Assume the **L** sitting position with your legs in a wide stride; then pull your legs together and then apart again. Use both small and large leg movements.

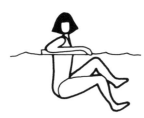

*BICYCLE   In a "chair" position, slowly move your legs in a bicycle motion to the front. This exercise may also be performed on each side.

96

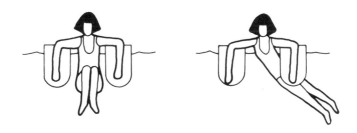

KNEE TO CHEST EXTENSION

Starting with your knees drawn into your chest, rotate your body and shoot your legs underneath one kickboard. Repeat to the opposite side. Make sure the abdominals are contracted.

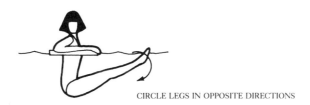

CIRCLE LEGS IN OPPOSITE DIRECTIONS

BUTTERFLY

In an **L** sitting position, lift your legs to the surface of the water and then swing them in a butterfly motion, moving your legs out, around, down, and back to the surface.

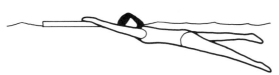

*KICKS

Holding one kickboard in front of your body, perform any of the swimming kicks, flutter, frog, or scissors.

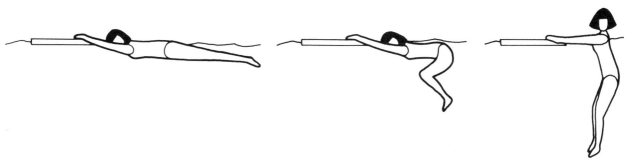

GLIDE AND JACKKNIFE DOWN

Holding one kickboard in front of your body, push off with both feet. Glide on the water; then bring your knees to your chest and then straight down to a standing position. Return to the starting position and repeat 8 times.

97

The Eat Rich/ Stay Thin Diet

Eat rich, stay thin. It sounds almost too good to be true, but guests at Palm-Aire are treated every day to elegant menus that still allow them to lose weight, and you can share the secrets that make it possible at home.

When waistbands grow snug and we're unhappy with the bodies we see in the mirror, the most common reaction is to latch onto the latest fad diet and hope for an instant cure. Diets are so much a part of the American mentality that you can nearly always find one on the best-seller list. Usually, there's a different one every year. That alone ought to tell us something.

We keep seeking new magic formulas, but, in truth, every fad diet is doomed to fail. The very notion of going "on" a diet implies that you will go off it again. Most fad diets are based on deprivation, and most individuals are not going to continue to deprive themselves purposely for very long.

That is why fad diets are futile. As we've seen, they simply slow down the metabolism as the body learns to get along with less fuel, ensuring that you will put on pounds even faster than usual once you go back to a normal eating pattern.

The only eating plan that works in the long run is not a temporary diet, which keeps you thinking about what you *can't* eat, but a permanent way of planning well-balanced menus that concentrate on what you *can* and should be eating to lose weight without feeling deprived.

So at Palm-Aire we say *don't* diet. The Palm-Aire Plan is not based on doing without. Instead, it is a program of sound nutrition know-how and creative menu planning that will produce effective weight loss now, and weight maintenance forever.

When you read the recipe section at the end of this book, you will see that it includes such treats as lasagna, soufflés, bran muffins, seafood marinara, stuffed chicken, veal florentine, and chicken liver pâté, hardly the kind of food to make you feel cheated, and not at all the menus you'd expect to take off weight! Yet, you can and will lose weight on this food plan, which is based on 800 to 1,000 calories daily. You will lose 3 to 5 pounds this week and, if you continue to follow this eating pattern, you will steadily take off 1 to 2 pounds a week, without drastically slowing your metabolism. Couple wise planning and eating with regular exercise that speeds up the body's ability to burn calories, and you will lose weight even faster.

There is no hocus-pocus in the Palm-Aire meal plan, just common sense plus imagination and culinary know-how. A vital part of the Plan is portion control, learning to be satisfied with less when you eat. The stomach is actually an organ no bigger than a fist. It expands as you eat, and, if you eat a lot, it becomes used to expanding a lot. But you can quickly change what it takes to make your stomach feel full. Within a short time, your body will adjust to reduced portions, and you will find you are not only satisfied with less but actually feel uncomfortable when you overeat.

Spa guests are often amazed at how full they feel after a Spa meal. This is because the Palm-Aire menu offers meals made up of several courses, guaranteed to satisfy your psychological hunger for a variety of tastes and textures. After a fruit cup or a cup of broth and a healthy portion of salad, a smaller main course can seem quite filling. Soup is especially helpful at the start of a meal, because the warmth raises the internal body temperature and helps shut down hunger.

No one need leave the table feeling denied because they could not have dessert. The sweet taste at the end of the meal craved by everyone does not have to come from high-calorie cakes and pies. You'll find many clever, light, low-calorie dessert recipes on your Spa menu.

The next Spa secret you'll learn is how to substitute tasty low-calorie ingredients for the fattening ingredients normally used in cooking. There are many painless ways to cut your calorie consumption. If you learn the calorie counts of different foods, you'll discover that a cup of green peas contains 110 calories, while the same amount of green beans has only 25. A cup of plain lowfat yogurt substituted for a cup of sour cream in a dip saves 375 calories. Nonstick pots and pans and no-stick vegetable cooking spray, will save you 100 calories for every pat of butter or margarine you don't use. Even small substitutions can total up to a savings of many calories over the course of a week.

Consider that an extra 100 calories a day above what your body needs will result in a gain of about 10 pounds over a year. Consider that an average woman who uses up 1,200 calories daily will lose 12 pounds in one year if she cuts just 120 calories a day. You can easily see that small savings can add up to a large difference. Here are some other calorie-saving examples:

Substitutions	Calories saved
1 cup 1% lowfat milk for 1 cup whole milk	50
1 cup 1% lowfat creamed cottage cheese for 1 cup regular creamed cottage cheese	70
2 tablespoons grated Parmesan cheese for 1 ounce Cheddar	60
1 ounce mozzarella for 1 ounce American cheese	28
1 sandwich-size pita bread for 2 slices regular bread	90
1 cup bouillon from a cube instead of 1 cup canned chicken noodle soup	236
1 glass of wine for 1 mixed cocktail	55
2 egg whites for 1 egg yolk (in some recipes)	63
Puréed fresh fruit for syrup or jelly on toast or pancakes	30

Refer often to the calorie chart at the end of this book to become familiar with foods that offer you the most eating pleasure and variety with the least number of calories.

You'll note that the charts tell you something about each food besides the number of calories it contains. The amounts noted for protein, fat, and carbohydrates measure the three basic nutrients that account for the calories in food. The body needs each one of them to function properly. One reason that fad diets are hard to stay with is because the body becomes fatigued if it does not get all the nutrients it needs. Another is that you begin psychologically to feel deprived if your diet lacks variety.

Protein-rich foods, such as meat, eggs, cheese, milk, grains, and legumes (soy and kidney beans, and the like), are necessary for maintaining the body's bones, muscles, and organs. Fat, obtained mainly from oil, butter, nuts, whole milk products, and fatty meats, provides long-term stored energy. Fat is the most concentrated source of energy, *and* as the name suggests, it is the most fattening, the highest in calories.

Carbohydrates provide immediate energy by supplying blood sugar to the central nervous system and the brain. They come in two categories, however. Complex carbohydrates are also known as "natural" carbohydrates, because they are found in natural foods, such as vegetables, fruits, and whole cereal grains. These are foods relatively low in calories and rich in fiber; they help to keep the digestive system functioning well. Fruits and vegetables also contain a good amount of water, which makes them more filling, helping to curb the appetite.

Refined or "simple" carbohydrates, such as refined sugar, have higher calorie counts. Because there is sugar in sweets, such as cakes and other desserts that are high in calories but low in nutrients, these are the foods that have what are sometimes referred to as "empty calories."

Unfortunately, the deserved reputation of refined carbohydrates as "fattening" is often mistakenly carried over to natural carbohydrates. Many popular slimming diets are high protein–low carbohydrate in makeup. They appear to take a lot of weight off you in a hurry, partly because many carbohydrates contain a lot of water, but the good news you see on the scale represents a weight loss that is mostly water as well. The pounds will return as soon as you return to the healthy balanced diet your body needs.

Nor does this type of diet give your body the nutrients it needs to stay well and maintain energy. The ideal proportions of a healthy diet are high in carbohydrates—55 to 65 percent carbohydrate, with 10 to 15 percent protein and 25 to 35 percent fat.

Studies show that for most of us the real culprit in weight control is not carbohydrates but fat. The average American diet consists of 40 to 45 percent fat, far more than we require. Since fat contains about 9 calories per gram, while carbohydrates contain about 4 calories per gram, it is easy to see that an ounce of fat is equal to more than double the calories of a comparable amount of carbohydrates. It's not a slice of bread that will add damaging pounds, but the butter you spread on it!

Carbohydrates are valuable also because they act as kindling, the preliminary energy the body needs to start burning fat. Like kindling, they work best if used a little at a time. Ideally, we should eat more complex carbohydrates—pasta, potatoes, whole grain bread, fruits, and vegetables—and evenly space the size and frequency of our meals and healthful snacks throughout the day, rather than concentrating on three heavy meals.

American eating habits, which tend to progress during the day from a small breakfast to a medium lunch to a large dinner run exactly counter to the body's energy pattern. We load up on calories at the end of the day just as the body is winding down its activities. A small carbohydrate snack in midmorning and midafternoon can curb your appetite just enough so that you will be satisfied with less at lunch and dinner and help you to maintain a higher energy level as well.

Because fat is so packed with calories, a significant way to make meals less fattening lies in reducing or eliminating fat-laden foods, such as butter, margarine, oil, mayonnaise, and oil-based salad dressings. You'll notice that many of the Spa recipes use broth or fruit juice in place of oil or butter for sautéing. The results are absolutely delicious. Broth can also be thickened with arrowroot, instead of the usual butter-flour roux, for a tasty sauce. And every day there are more brands of reduced oil salad dressings and mayonnaise on the grocery shelves.

We have all been made aware of the importance of cutting back on excess cholesterol, which is found primarily in saturated fats in foods such as meat, eggs, and dairy products. Cholesterol can cause the accumulation of fatty deposits in the arteries (plaque), which hamper free circulation of the blood and increase the risk of heart disease. It has been indicated as a possible factor in many other diseases as well. Because nutritious protein-rich foods the body needs to build strong bones, such as meats and dairy products, also contain cholesterol, it should not be eliminated entirely in a well-balanced eating plan; instead, it should be used creatively in smaller quantities. The Palm-Aire food plan favors low-fat and low-calorie protein sources, such as fish and skinless chicken. You may change your food choices on your own, too, when you learn that an 8-ounce rib-eye steak contains the fat equivalent of *15* pats of butter!

But you don't have to give up meat entirely. There are countless ways to use small amounts of meat to balance the diet and please the palate. One Spa "secret" is to slice meat or chicken thinly and add lots of vegetables, and a portion of pasta or rice, to provide tasty healthy bulk that leaves you feeling full and satisfied after a light, healthy dinner. Dishes along these lines give you the amount of protein you require and still let you cut down on calories and fat. Broiled shish kabob with small chunks of meat alternating with crunchy vegetables, served on rice is another excellent example of calorie- and cholesterol-conscious recipes that offer ample protein.

A secondary plus in cutting down on protein is that excess protein is stored by the body as fat; eating smaller portions will also help to control fat.

Salt, which has been linked to high blood pressure, and which encourages the body to retain fluids, is eliminated as a seasoning in the Palm-Aire Plan. Learning how to make and use delicious herb seasonings the Palm-Aire way with dill, tarragon, sage, or basil, or seasoning your food with garlic, onion, and lemon juice to take the place of salt, will help you create dishes that contribute to a healthier diet without sacrificing full taste pleasure at mealtime. A vegetable seasoning product such as Mrs. Dash can take its place next to the pepper shaker on your table, just as at Palm-Aire. It's a great flavor enhancer, perfect for those who find it hard to break the habit of adding seasoning to their food.

If you don't have high blood pressure, you needn't worry that you are depleting your body of necessary salt on this food plan. Salt is found in overabundance in so many prepared foods—mustard, ketchup, canned tomato juice, canned tomato sauce, and bouillon, just to name a few—that you will have little difficulty getting your daily requirement. By cutting back when you cook, you will simply avoid taking in far more salt than your body needs.

Only decaffeinated coffee and herbal tea are included in the Palm-Aire food plan, discouraging the use of artificial stimulants and encouraging you to develop naturally through exercise the stimulation your body needs. Many people are surprised at how little they miss the caffeine they thought they could not do without.

As for calorie-rich sugar, every time you eliminate ¼ cup, you save 200 calories. In most recipes, you can cut back one-third on the sugar called for, and easily enhance the taste with added spices like cinnamon and nutmeg, or vanilla or almond extract. Experiment to find a reduced sugar level that pleases your palate. Even icing can be replaced with a dusting of confectioners sugar. And you can make yummy, "sinful-tasting" desserts with many naturally sweet fruits like pears, bananas, and apples—delicious taste treats without any added sugar! Puréed fresh fruits are a tasty low-calorie replacement for breakfast jams and jellies as well.

Non-nutritive chemically sweetened soft drinks are not forbidden at Palm-Aire, but they are discouraged. Though they are artificially sweetened and contain no calories, they perpetuate a taste for sweets, and prevent you from trying to re-educate those taste buds.

One liquid that *is* strongly recommended is water. Good old H_2O. The reason 8 glasses of water each day is recommended is because the body needs water to operate its systems at top efficiency, and the more efficiently the body operates, the better for your health. Water has another distinct advantage. It helps to fill you up, adding only a single calorie!

As for vitamins, a daily multivitamin is a healthy safeguard while you are on a reduced-calorie food plan, but if you follow the Palm-Aire eating philosophy, which advocates a nutritionally balanced diet, you should get all the vitamins you need without a supplement.

Whittling down sugar, sodium, and fat in your food will help whittle away your waistline and need not make your meals any less tasty. Your palate will soon adapt to these lighter tastes, and you will find that you actually prefer them. You will certainly not miss the bloated feeling after meals that comes from an overly rich diet.

You will enjoy finding a wonderful, healthful new way of cooking with Spa-tested recipes that let you serve elegant meals and still lose weight. The recipe section at the end of this book contains enough recipes for 7 full days of menus, all within your calorie limits.

Equally important, you will be able to experiment and create your own original, delicious low-calorie dishes by learning the secrets of healthier meal planning that these menus can teach you.

One perennial problem that presents itself when you are watching your weight is eating out. Many of the principles you'll be practicing in your kitchen on the Palm-Aire Plan can be carried over to dining out in restaurants. Order clear soup and a big salad with just a little bit of dressing; then eat only half your main course, and you can order almost anything on a menu occasionally without doing serious damage.

At lunch hour, beware of restaurants offering a "diet special." It often consists of a burger, cottage cheese, and a canned peach, high in fat and sugar and far from low calorie! A chef's salad is also deceptive. Ham and cheese and salad dressing are all high in fat. You're far better off ordering a turkey sandwich on whole wheat bread with lettuce and tomato—just have them hold the mayo.

When you go out for dinner, give some thought to the kind of restaurant you choose. If you go to a steak house or a French restaurant specializing in rich sauces, you have little chance of holding down the calories. Italian, Japanese, and Chinese restaurants are better bets. They offer the possibility of entrées built around carbohydrates, such as pasta or rice, that use small amounts of proteins like meat, fish, or chicken. If you order dishes like chicken chow mein or shrimp marinara, you can enjoy your meal with a minimum of damage to your waistline. Wherever you dine, fish is always a dependable low-calorie choice—as long as it isn't swimming in rich sauce!

You'll find the Palm-Aire Plan allows you to have many delicious foods whether you are dining in or out. But the big question most of us have to face before we are ready to go ahead and succeed in changing our eating habits is *why* we have been eating more than our bodies need in the first place.

Breaking Bad Habits

You know you need to take off some weight: Waistbands that don't quite close and excess padding around the hips are unmistakable signs. Yet here you are again, heading for the kitchen to raid the cookie jar and the ice cream carton.

What is it that makes so many of us continue to overeat, even when we don't like the image that looks back at us from the mirror?

It is not only because we feel hungry. Seventy-five percent of our eating is directed strictly by the mind. Eating is tied into so many emotions and habits that is is hard to recognize all of our own motivations.

Some of our "fat habits" are learned from childhood. It's less a matter of genes than habit. Growing up accustomed to a starchy, fat-laden, or overabundant diet instills a taste for fattening food and large portions that carries over into adulthood. If you were not encouraged to be active when you were young, your metabolism has likely grown sluggish, making it easier for you to gain weight. The way you learned to eat—big meals instead of light ones, gobbling food down so that you consume more instead of savoring it slowly and eating less—also may have taught you fattening habits.

Age is another factor. Your body burns calories in two ways, through exercise and through natural and conditioned changes in metabolism, the internal functions that keep the body going. The metabolism slows down 2 percent every decade after age thirty-five. Few people increase their activity to make up that deficit over the years; it's more likely that we decrease exercising. That's why we gain weight more readily with age even though our diets may not change.

But that doesn't mean that staying overweight is inevitable. Many of the habits that lead to gaining weight are learned, and can be just as easily unlearned. If you recognize these destructive patterns, you have a head start on changing them.

You've already learned the importance of becoming more active in order to burn more calories. There's more to learn! If you are overeating as well as underexercising now, one of the most productive things you can do is to keep a food diary for a week or two, recording when and where and what you eat—and how you feel each time you eat. Then make a list of "When I eat" and "When I don't eat" and compare them.

Most of us do a lot of unnecessary eating that has little to do with hunger. If you concentrate on changing the situations that tempt you to eat, finding substitute satisfactions for foods, you will have made real headway in cutting calories even before you make any change in the foods you eat. Here's a suggested list of entries for your own food diary:

SAMPLE FOOD DIARY

Time	Date	Location	Activity	Alone?	Reason for eating	Food eaten
10:00 A.M.	6/5	office	phone calls	yes	bored and stressed	buttered roll coffee
12:30 P.M.	6/5	pizza place	social lunch	no	lunch out	3 slices pizza, Tab
5:30 P.M.	6/5	restaurant	party for business	no	social (nervous)	2 gin and tonics, chips, crudités, cheese and crackers

7:30 P.M.	6/5	home	dinner	yes	dinner	broiled chicken, salad and dressing, iced tea, peach
9:30 P.M.	6/5	home	watching TV	yes	restless	6 cookies

You'll probably recognize certain "eating cues"—boredom, anger, tension, nervous energy—that lead you to foods you don't really need. Having spotted them, you need to work on substitute reactions—alternate things to do when the urge to eat strikes.

For example, if anger makes you turn to food for consolation, try to find another way to work out your feelings. Call a friend and talk the problem out, write your feelings down, or work the anger off by punching your pillow, hitting golf balls or tennis balls, or running around the block.

If boredom is the culprit, get busy: Clean a closet, work on a photo album, tackle a problem task, or go out and take a walk. Keep a list of undone chores to attack when the boredom bug bites.

When you feel sad or tense, instead of consoling yourself with sweets, talk to a friend, treat yourself to something (not edible!) you really like, or try some of the relaxation techniques in the "Stress and De-Stress" chapter.

You get the idea: Learn to seek satisfaction that is unrelated to food.

Simple changes in the way you eat can also help you cut calories. Eating slowly will make you eat less. It takes 20 minutes for your stomach to signal your brain that you have had enough to eat. If you eat too quickly, you will have already overeaten before your brain gets the message.

Slowing down also means you will pay more attention to how food tastes, and you will enjoy your food more—that helps you to finish your meals feeling full and more satisfied having eaten less.

An important Spa technique you can use easily at home is to make mealtime more special. You'll be amazed how this simple strategy can help you lose weight without feeling deprived. Plan every meal to *feel* special, no matter how few the calories. At breakfast, why not treat yourself to exotic fresh fruit like papaya or kiwi (often even lower in calories yet more filling than juice) and a special low-calorie omelet or the crêpes you will find in the Palm-Aire Plan recipe list? For lunch and dinner, always include several courses—soup, salad, and dessert, as well as the main course—and try to dine in the same leisurely, pleasant way you would if you were eating in a fine restaurant. Light the candles at dinner. Use the good dishes. Make your table festive, your plate attractive and appealing, and your low-calorie menu as tempting as you know how. Be creative. Get involved in the presentation as well as the preparation of your meals.

You may need to make a special effort to create pleasant ambience if you are eating alone. It's all too easy to eat in a hurry or to distract yourself with a book or TV instead of paying attention to your food, which often leads to overeating, almost without your realizing what you are doing.

There are a number of other eating patterns you can alter and new good habits you can form that will aid you in your weight loss program. Here are a number of proven tips passed along at Palm-Aire:

1. *When you eat, do nothing else but eat.* Sit down at the table in the kitchen or dining room or in a restaurant. It's easy to lose track of how much you eat when your nose is in a book, your mind is on your chores, or your eyes are on the typewriter or a television screen. Don't walk around the house munching, or snack in front of the TV, or at your desk.

2. *Make each meal last longer.* Try to take at least 20 minutes for a meal. Plan several courses. Chew each mouthful of food carefully. Put your fork down between bites to slow you down. If you take your time, you will feel much more satisfied when you are done.

3. *Make a habit of always leaving some food on your plate.* The "clean plate club" leads to automatic eating even after you are no longer hungry, especially in restaurants where portions are often too large. At home, you can avoid leaving the leftovers around to tempt you by freezing any extras immediately.

4. *When your main course is finished, take a break.* Clear the table, do the dishes, have coffee or tea. Only after your beverage is finished should you ask yourself if you really want dessert. Don't just serve it automatically. Even if you do eat it, it's a good idea to save your dessert for later, and have it as a midevening snack.

5. *Cut down on serving sizes.* Fool yourself into forgetting that your portions are smaller than they used to be. Be artistic. Space food attractively on the plate and use parsley, lemon wedges, or other garnishes to fill in the empty spaces. Or, you can simply use smaller dishes. At Palm-Aire, dinner often arrives on a regular-size dinner plate. On top of the plate is a

pretty paper doily—and on top of the doily is a smaller glass plate containing the entrée.

6. *Don't bring extra food to the table*. Dish out servings right from the stove instead of placing the serving dishes on the table, where second helpings are all too readily available.

7. *Avoid temptation*. Don't bring problem foods into the house: If you have them, at some point you are probably going to eat them. Shop only from a list and not on impulse. Avoid foods that are easy to grab and eat—unless they are celery or carrot sticks. Put fattening food in containers you can't see through or wrap them in aluminum foil. And *never* leave out dishes of candy or nuts.

8. *Post a list of activities to divert your attention when the urge to snack strikes*. Drink a healthy glass of water or a cup of herbal tea, take a walk or a run up and down the stairs, make a phone call—anything will do as long as it takes your mind off food.

9. *Have only low-calorie snacks on hand, just in case your willpower fails*. The snacking habit dies hard, so if you must indulge yourself occasionally, do so with the least amount of damage. Slice those carrot and celery sticks and keep them in the refrigerator in a cup of cold water, ready to grab instead of fattening cookies. Pop up a batch of unbuttered popcorn, which has only a fraction of the calories of potato or corn chips. It's especially helpful to have low-calorie alternatives on hand to munch during a cocktail hour to take the place of more fattening munchables.

10. *Make a list of things other than food that can serve as a reward or a solace*. Break the habit of using food to feed your emotions. Buy yourself a present, take in a movie or play, call a friend long distance, or take a long, luxurious bubble bath—anything that doesn't add up to calories.

11. *Control binging*. No one is likely to stay on an eating plan that never allows for an ice cream cone, a chocolate bar, or a cookie. By all means, give yourself an occasional treat, but don't let it turn into a binge. Go out for a single ice cream cone instead of bringing home half a gallon of ice cream. Once you have it, you'll probably end up eating it: We all share that perverse habit of deciding to finish off the container so it won't be around to tempt us anymore. Buy a cookie or two at the bakery to avoid eating a whole box of Oreos or Fig Newtons at home. Binging is almost always done in private where nobody is watching. Therefore, it's safer to have your treats in public.

12. *Praise yourself as much for habit changes as for actual weight loss.* Give yourself rewards for progress, because eventually it *will* show up on the scale.

Changing some of your eating habits can help you cut down on food, but according to the nutritionists at Palm-Aire, the most difficult thing to change is your attitude. Don't ignore the psychology of dieting. The idea of dieting is a negative one. It implies you must be perfect or you won't get results. But everyone slips when they try to change long-accustomed ways, including eating habits. Too many people think only about their failures and what they are missing in the course of losing weight. They get discouraged and quit, instead of accepting human nature and picking up where they left off after a lapse.

To expect perfection is unrealistic. You don't have to be perfect to lose weight. The secret is eating well *most* of the time, and eating "bad" foods infrequently and in small amounts. If you can satisfy the small cravings, you're less likely to binge.

The Palm-Aire Plan menu is proof that if you pay attention to preparing particularly tasty low-calorie dishes while you are trying to lose weight, you can avoid still another dieting pitfall—that of dwelling on what you are not supposed to eat. Why not think hard about what you *can* have? Build a repertoire of tasty healthful recipes such as the ones you will use this week, dishes you can look forward to cooking and eating. Think about your low-calorie meals positively, and you will increase the likelihood of success in changing your eating habits.

Visual rehearsing is a tactic that can also help you stick to a better eating and exercise regimen. Many successful people have used visualization to attain a variety of goals. Some athletes report that they imagine themselves at peak performance before they actually compete. You can use this same strategy to help yourself succeed in shaping up. Instead of looking at yourself in the mirror and feeling discouraged by your failings, close your eyes and imagine yourself becoming active and slim. Really try to imagine how you will look, feel, and behave as a thin person, the clothes you will wear, the new activities you will try. Such pleasant daydreaming can provide the determination you need to make these dreams come true.

Every day and in every way you can discover things to help change your old attitudes—and your old self-image. Look for little ways to become more active. Use the stairs instead of the elevator. Walk to work or ride your bike to the neighborhood stores instead of driving the car or taking the bus. You'll not only burn calories but you will reinforce your new image of yourself as a more active person.

Along with your own attitudes, you will have to contend with family and friends, who may unwittingly make it harder for you to lose weight. Nobody operates in a vacuum. You can't expect others to change their perception of you or to change their own ways just because *you* are doing so. If your family or your friends feel threatened or uncomfortable with your new fitness habits, they can undermine your efforts. So, don't try to force others to diet or exercise with you. Instead, talk to the key people in your life: Explain the Spa Plan, what you are trying to accomplish, and why it is important to you, and ask them for their support.

Above all, get rid of that "all or nothing" mentality that brands you a failure unless you stick to your plan 100 percent. Vowing you will *never* snack again or promising to exercise twice a day for the rest of your life is unrealistic and will only guarantee a sense of defeat when you can't measure up. Give yourself due credit for your successes, and remember that backsliding is only temporary—and only human.

Learn to look for the positive, give yourself a pat instead of a kick; it's all part of feeling better about yourself, and that's one of the primary goals of the Palm-Aire Plan. Taking better care of your body is a big step in the right direction.

Making the Most of Yourself

From a glowing complexion to a glossy pedicure, a well-cared-for body is a guaranteed ego-booster. Your grooming reflects to the world how you feel about yourself—and looking your best, in turn, makes you feel even better about yourself.

If you have been too busy or too discouraged to take proper care of your grooming needs recently, you'll find that just one week of attention can work minor miracles, providing a special lift every time you look into the mirror. And nowhere can you see a more dramatic change for the better than where it matters most—your own face.

BEST FACE FORWARD

Whether you are a movie star or a matron, slim or stocky, old or young, one of the first things people notice about you is your complexion. No change can subtract years from your appearance as quickly as fresher, smoother skin.

Palm-Aire's secret to a lovelier complexion is simply to

help the skin do what it does naturally—renew itself every single day. By understanding and working with this remarkable process of renewal, you will soon be rewarded with a fresher, healthier glow.

If you could look at your skin through a microscope, you would see that this thin, fragile membrane is composed of several distinct layers, with an extra layer of fat beneath to provide a cushion and give the skin a springy, youthful texture. Two of these layers are of special importance in skin care.

The deepest skin layer, the dermis, is made of tough connective tissues, elastin and collagen, which account for the skin's elasticity. This layer also contains the sweat and sebaceous glands. Sebaceous glands produce an oil called *sebum* and send it to the surface through the pores, where it combines with the moisture from the sweat glands to produce a product known as the *acid mantle*. It is this acid mantle that keeps the skin supple and soft.

The layer of skin we see, the epidermis, actually has several sublayers. The minuscule cells that make up the skin's surface begin forming at the deepest of these layers and work their way up. Cells lose moisture on the way, and by the time they reach the surface, they have dried up and their life span is over, a process that takes only about 28 days. These cells are so minute and so numerous that newer cells pushing their way up will slough off old ones at a rate of several million a day.

How can we help the skin in its work? First, by taking care to use gentle products that will not disturb the acid mantle. Next, by helping to clear away the top layer of dead cell tissue, which can hide the healthy glow of the newer cells lying just underneath. These two goals can be achieved at the same time with a luxurious facial, which also stimulates circulation, relieves tension, and leaves you looking younger and feeling better all over. It's one of the real pleasures you can look forward to during your Palm-Aire Spa week.

But facials are not a substitute for daily care. The most important thing you can do for your skin is to keep it absolutely clean every single day. It should be cleansed every morning and every night without fail. The technique for cleansing is simple, though it may vary somewhat according to your skin type—oily, dry, or normal. Because few people have skin that is all one type, different portions of your face may need different kinds of care.

The following are the basic steps to proper daily skin care:

You will need: *Creamy liquid cleanser   Skin toner*
                   Large roll of cotton   Moisturizer

STEP 1: CLEANSE. The most effective way to cleanse the skin is with a gentle, milky liquid cleanser with an oil and water base. The oil speeds the cleansing process and the water assures that a damp cotton pad is all you need to remove the cleanser when its job is done. Do *not* rub sensitive facial skin with a face cloth. Saturate wads of cotton and use them to apply the cleanser to your face with firm upward strokes; use as many pieces of cotton as necessary to remove all the grime. Take a few extra minutes to work your fingers upward and inward in a massaging motion to help keep wrinkles away.

Never use soap on dry skin. If you have a normal or oily complexion, and simply do not feel clean unless you use soap, choose a brand with the lowest possible alkaline content. Alkalines strip away the skin's natural acid mantle and upset its chemical balance.

If you have oily skin, you may use beauty grains every few days to add a slightly abrasive cleaning action in areas with enlarged pores. If you have sensitive skin or skin with broken capillaries, avoid abrasive cleansing and water that is either very hot or very cold; lukewarm is best.

STEP 2: TONE. Washing should be followed by the application of toning lotion, which cools the skin with an evaporating effect, temporarily causing muscles to contract and pores to appear smaller. Apply toner with wet cotton pads that have had excess water squeezed out. Blot toner quickly with tissues to prevent further evaporation that can dry the skin.

Toning is refreshing and removes any traces of grease left on the skin. There are several kinds of products for this purpose—fresheners, toners, clarifying lotions, and astringents. Fresheners are the mildest and often contain lemon juice or citric acid to restore the acid balance of the skin after washing. Toners and clarifying lotions contain alcohol, which makes them more drying and abrasive. Astringents are harshest of all; they have a high percentage of alcohol, which makes them extremely drying to the skin. They should be used only on very oily complexions.

STEP 3: MOISTURIZE. Moisturizers cannot actually put moisture into the skin—that is done only from within. What they do is help to hold moisture in, plumping up the cells and making the skin look softer in the process. There are oil-based emulsions for dry skin and lighter preparations with water bases for those who do not need extra oil. You can usually tell the difference by the texture of the lotion or cream. All types work most efficiently when applied to damp skin. Use moisturizer in the morning and as a base under makeup. Do not apply moisturizer as a night cream; while it holds in moisture, it also blocks pores. Choose a cream formulated for night use instead.

NIGHT SKIN CARE

Remove all makeup, and cleanse and tone, following the first two steps above. Use gentle products especially made for removing eye makeup.

STEP 1: LUBRICATE. Do not be misled by products that promise to nourish your skin. No miracle ingredient can do that because the skin can be nourished only from within. A healthy complexion is simply evidence of a healthy well-balanced diet, the best gift you can give to your skin.

However, if your skin is dry, a night cream can help lubricate the top layer. Look for creams that contain natural animal or vegetable oils and vitamins beneficial to the skin, such as vitamins A, E, or H (biotin).

STEP 2: MASSAGE. After you apply cream, stroke your face lightly with your fingertips several times, using long, slow, upward strokes from neck to scalp. Massage stimulates the nerve endings under the skin and helps improve the circulation and texture of dry or aging skin.

When it comes to choosing products to cleanse and care for your skin, ingredients and personal preferences are more important than brand names. Learn to read labels to make sure you know the kind of base from which each product is made. It is counterproductive, for example, to use a mild cleansing cream for dry skin and then follow it with a drying alcohol-based toner. You may find it helpful to consult a professional cosmetician or a dermatologist about products that are beneficial for your particular skin type.

Experiment to find a brand of cosmetics that pleases you, and as the Palm-Aire cosmeticians advise, use the entire line, as the different products will contain compatible ingredients. However, they also note that it is good to change brands periodically, because, after a while, your skin becomes immune to ingredients applied frequently and will respond better to a new formula.

THE EXTRA STEP: EXFOLIATION

There is one valuable additional step in skin care that makes a glowing difference. Old cells remaining on the surface of the skin tend to give your face a dull finish. Removing this outer layer of dead cells with the gentle stimulation of exfoliation reveals the finer, softer layer underneath.

Unless you have very dry skin, an exfoliating cleansing with gentle beauty grains should be done once a week. Use a commercial preparation or make your own by mixing cornmeal with a facial moisturizer.

Another beneficial kind of exfoliation is a facial mask. It seals moisture into the skin and lifts off surface cells when it is removed. A mask has many other benefits as well. It relaxes, tones, brightens, lightens, firms, refines, and refreshes the skin. Anyone over the age of thirteen can benefit from using a mask every week.

THE ULTIMATE TREATMENT: FACIALS

A facial treatment combines the use of a mask with gentle, thorough cleaning, creaming, and facial massage. It is a totally luxurious and rejuvenating experience. Facials cannot actually erase wrinkles or restore lost skin tone. They can't make you young again, but they definitely *can* make you look and feel that way! Facials are one of the special pleasures of a spa visit, and can be one of the highlights of your Spa week at home as well.

HOW TO GIVE YOURSELF A FACIAL

You will need:
Cleansing products (liquid cleanser, cotton, eye makeup remover, etc.)
Cleansing granules (bought or homemade)
Lubricating skin cream
Skin freshener
Hand cream
Skin mask (a commercial product or a natural mask—see recipes below)
Pure water in an atomizer

1. Pull your hair back from your face with a headband or clips.

2. Cleanse your skin thoroughly (as directed on page 117).

3. Use granules to scrub gently and deeply in areas that tend to collect blackheads, such as the sides of your nose, the inner portion of your chin, and the area of your brow between your eyes. (Do not use grains over skin with broken capillaries.)

4. Splash the granules away with tepid water; pat your skin dry with tissues.

5. Apply an eye cream to soften tiny lines under your eyes. (Honey is a natural softener that performs very well here.)

6. Apply a layer of skin cream on your neck; saturate a tissue with astringent or witch hazel and drape it around your neck over the cream;

then wring dry a hot moist towel (as hot as you can stand it) and wrap it around your neck as a compress.

7. Apply a facial mask evenly over all of your face, except the area around your eyes. Do this in front of the mirror to be sure you cover your face thoroughly. Use any of the many commercial masks available or one of the following natural recipes.

8. Take the phone off the hook, cover your hands with hand cream, lie down, and close your eyes. Let the mask work for 10 to 20 minutes, as directed.

9. Remove the towel, tissue, and cream from your neck; then remove the mask with cotton that has been dampened in tepid water.

10. Pat on freshener with moist cotton pads.

11. Spray your face with a pure water, such as Evian, and pat it into your skin with a tissue.

12. Apply moisturizer to seal moisture into your skin.

Here are some suggested ingredients for natural masks:

Beaten egg whites (egg whites can also be used occasionally around the eyes to contract lines temporarily)
Evaporated milk mixed with egg yolk
Lemon juice mixed with baking soda and cream
Lemon juice mixed with egg whites
Lemon juice mixed with plain yogurt
2 ounces of buttermilk mixed with 2 tablespoons of whole wheat flour
Dried brewer's yeast mixed with warm distilled water and 2 tablespoons of milk (for this mask, cover your face with cheesecloth and then apply the mixture; cover with a towel dipped in powdered milk reconstituted with distilled water)

A WORD ABOUT AGING

As the years go by, the sebaceous glands shrink in size and produce less oil, so that skin tends to become dryer with age. Your skin care routine should change accordingly. By the time you reach the age of thirty, it is wise to use a good moisturizer daily to help hold in moisture and keep the skin supple. By forty, every skin care product you use should moisturize and soften. Moisturizers are essential by day and a rich cream should be used at night. Use a room humidifier in winter to be kind to your skin and to avoid the drying effects of overheated rooms.

The skin's rate of cell division and replacement also falls off after the age of thirty-five. As your skin becomes less efficient in replacing old cells with new, exfoliation to remove dead surface cells becomes more important than ever to ensure that the texture of your skin remains clear, smooth, and glowing. Facial masks are the gentlest way to remove dead skin cells from the surface.

Time also takes its toll on the collagen and elastin fibers of the skin. Like rubber bands that have been stretched too much, they tend to lose their elasticity, resulting in sagging, wrinkling, and loss of skin tone. You cannot stop the clock to stop wrinkles from forming, but you definitely can delay and minimize them.

The single most important thing you can do to ward off wrinkles is to avoid the sun. The damage caused by sun is cumulative. But even if you overexposed your skin in your younger years, you can prevent further damage by protecting it now.

Facial exercises may also help keep those lines from forming in common trouble spots like foreheads and around the mouth. Repeat these often:

1. Raise and lower your eyebrows to stretch the forehead and scalp. Raise your eyebrows upward and hold while you count to 5; rest and then repeat, pulling your eyebrows down for a count of 5.

2. Snarl.

3. Smile, first turning the corners of your mouth up toward your eyes; then turn them out toward your ears.

4. Stretch your tongue to the tip of your nose.

5. Pretend a bubble is in your mouth and roll it around in a circular motion.

It is believed that a rich supply of certain vitamins will benefit the skin:

- Vitamin A to help overcome dryness
- B complex to improve the function of the network of nerves beneath the skin
- E to help revitalize older skin
- K and F (linoleic acid) for skin disorders
- H (biotin) to help condition the skin and repair body tissues
- P (bioflavonoid) to help keep capillary walls flexible, avoiding broken capillaries

However, a well-balanced diet should give you all the vitamins you need, and supplements may not be required.

The overall health of your body is reflected in its outer layer, the skin. Eat well, get plenty of sleep, cut down on cigarettes and alcohol, and exercise regularly to keep your body's circulation—and your complexion—at its peak.

MORE SKIN CARE TIPS FROM PALM-AIRE

1. Some things that can damage your skin are:

- air pollution
- sun exposure
- lack of vitamins B and C
- improper skin care
- not enough deep cleaning
- use of alkaline soaps
- not enough fruit and vegetables in diet
- cigarette smoking
- too much alcohol

2. Things that can help your skin keep its natural loveliness are:

- good nutrition
- sun protection
- fresh air
- proper cleansing
- exercise
- relaxation
- daily skin care
- enough sleep, which is vitally important to allow the skin cells time to repair themselves
- plenty of water—8 glasses every day

3. Be fanatical about cleansing your face; it pays off.

4. Soap leaves a residue; it's best not to use it on your face.

5. Vaseline is an excellent, gentle, and inexpensive product for removing eye makeup.

6. An overnight paste of baking soda and water will dry up and draw out pimples.

7. Do not use a moisturizer under your eyes, particularly overnight. Mois-

turizers hold in water, tending to make eyes look puffy.

8. To tighten puffy skin beneath your eyes, apply cotton pads dipped in ice water, cold witch hazel, or cold tea.

9. For tired eyes, use cool tea bag packs. The tannic acid in tea not only reduces swelling but soothes red or bloodshot eyes.

10. Egg whites can be used to contract lines at the corners of your eyes temporarily, a good technique to use before a special date.

11. Do not use very cold or very hot water on skin with broken capillaries.

12. Remember to use protective lotion in harsh winter weather as well as in the sun.

13. Stay out of the sun—today's becoming tan may very well be tomorrow's ugly wrinkles.

CARE OF THE NECK

Cosmeticians know that the neck always reveals the true age of their clients. The neck ages prematurely, showing the effects of the years even faster than the face. A facial helps soften and beautify the neck, but there are other things you can do regularly to prevent the sagging skin that gives away your age. Try the following:

- Sleep without a pillow.
- Walk with your head held high, chin straight, and your shoulders down at normal level.
- Avoid deep armchairs, which encourage bad posture and break the line of your neck.
- Practice walking while you balance a book on your head.
- Perform these exercises every day to preserve the vitality and grace of your neck:

    Slowly incline your head from right to left and then forward and backward several times.
    Turn your head from right to left and then from left to right.
    Lean your head back, to the right, to the front, to the left, and then repeat.
    To combat the formation of a double chin, exert slow and progressive pressure on your bottom teeth with your tongue.

BODY LANGUAGE

A smooth, soft, and youthful body is a special personal pleasure. The Salt Glow/Loofah Scrub is one of the most popular services at Palm-Aire, a soothing and luxurious treatment that cleans, tingles, and leaves the body feeling baby-soft. And it is one of the easiest beauty procedures to treat yourself to at home.

The loofah, actually the dried fruit of the loofah plant, is a natural sponge. Its firm network of fibers gives a stimulating massage, yet it is gentle enough for sensitive skin. The abrasive texture of the loofah acts as a skin conditioner, stimulating circulation and removing dead skin cells, which is as beneficial for the body as for the face. Like a facial, the result of a loofah scrub is smoother, more glowing skin. You can purchase a loofah mitt in most department store cosmetic departments, many drug stores, and in most health food stores. Choose one with a convenient elastic band to hold it firmly on your hand.

HOW TO GIVE YOURSELF A SALT GLOW/LOOFAH SCRUB

You will need:
4 cups of kosher salt (you may use 2 cups of kosher and 2 cups of table salt)
2 ounces baby oil or avocado oil
Water
Bar of mild soap
Loofah mitt (if you cannot find one, use a natural sponge)

THE SALT GLOW. In a large mixing bowl, add enough water to the oil and salt to form a wet paste, and have it ready at the tub or shower. Wet your entire body with warm water. Take a handful of the Salt Glow mixture and apply it to your right foot and leg. Use up-and-down strokes and/or a circular motion to rub the mixture over your entire leg, front and back, and foot. Rub firmly but not so hard as to be uncomfortable. Add more mixture to your body as needed. Repeat the procedure on your left leg and foot and then move on to your left arm and underarm, right arm and underarm, abdomen, chest, back, and buttocks. (A circular motion feels quite comforting on the abdomen.)

There is no need to scrub hard. Avoid heavy pressure on varicose veins. Avoid the genital area and rub your breasts extra gently. Spend extra time on your elbows, fingers, knees, and toes, where scaly skin or calluses tend to collect. Do not use Salt Glow right after shaving or waxing. Avoid any areas where there are open or unhealed sores.

124

When you have scrubbed your entire body, rinse off thoroughly with warm water and proceed to the loofah scrub.

THE LOOFAH. Wet the loofah mitt well and rub a bar of gentle soap on it or dip the mitt in a soapy water solution. Following the same procedure as for the Salt Glow, generously apply the soap and water to each extremity and the torso. Massage your skin lightly in a circular motion until it blushes pink. When you are done, hang the loofah on end to drain and dry. It will last for several months before it loses its natural firmness.

Do not apply moisturizing lotion to the skin for at least a few hours. Your skin is now soft and clean from the bath oil and soap. Let the pores breathe.

Palm-Aire recommends a Salt Glow/Loofah every 4 weeks, and even more frequently on your feet. You can give yourself a loofah scrub in your bath or shower every day if you would like to keep your body tingly fresh and young. A loofah massage is a simple, natural way to stimulate circulation, soothe tired muscles, and relieve tension.

HOLDING HANDS

After your face, your hands are the most exposed and noticeable parts of your body—and no area indicates lack of care so obviously. Hands are delicate and quickly reflect the dehydrating effects of sun and harsh weather. Fortunately, a little regular attention can make a big difference in their condition, paying off with the smooth-feeling skin and shiny nails that reflect pride in your appearance.

Keep a bottle of hand cream or lotion right next to the sink and apply it every time you wash your hands, rubbing it into the cuticles as well. Within just one week you will see the change this undemanding routine will make.

Your fingernails also reflect the care they receive. With practice, you can learn to give yourself a professional-looking manicure that will reward you with hands pretty enough to show off. Here are instructions from the beauty salon at Palm-Aire for an outstanding home manicure.

You will need:
Emery boards
Orangewood stick
Cotton
Cuticle cream
Mild soap, warm water, small dish
Hand cream
Nail polish remover
Base coat polish
Nail polish
Top coat or hardener

1. Take off any old polish with remover-soaked cotton pads.

2. Use an emery board to create a squared or oval shape, working from the outside corners to the center of each nail. Never file deeply into the sides. Smooth ridged nails by buffing the tops gently with the fine side of the emery board.

3. Apply cuticle cream or sunflower oil to each nail, rubbing it into the cuticles.

4. Soak your hands in mild, soapy warm water for 3 minutes.

5. Clean beneath the nails with the pointed side of an orange stick wrapped lightly in cotton.

6. Wrap the wide end of the orange stick in a thin cotton layer, and carefully, with little pressure, push your cuticles back; then use a nail brush to scrub your nails clear of dead cuticle. *Never* use a steel implement—it damages the cuticles.

7. If necessary, use a cuticle trimmer to remove excess cuticle, but cut *only* dead tissue or stubborn pieces that stick up. It's far better to train the cuticle by gently pushing it back over a period of weeks.

8. Rub hand cream onto your hand and then your fingers, first pulling the finger joints outward and then pushing them back toward your knuckles. Massage the cream thoroughly into the backs and palms of your hands.

9. Use a cotton-coated orange stick soaked in polish remover to remove any oil left on your nails before you apply a base coat. A good polish base

is a very important foundation for a lasting manicure. If your nails are soft or brittle, use two coats of base. Stroke the base on the undersides of your nail tips for extra strength.

10. Apply two coats of color, allowing your nails to dry between coats. Keep handy an orange stick with a very thin cotton wrapping on the point; dip it in remover and carefully erase smudges as you apply polish.

11. Apply a protective top coat. If your nails are weak, use a clear nail hardener to strengthen them further.

12. Let your nails dry completely. After 15 minutes, you can set the polish by plunging your fingers into a bowl of ice water.

13. Apply follow-up coats of polish daily.

14. Remove all polish and repeat your manicure once a week.

PALM-AIRE'S SPECIAL HAND AND NAIL CARE HINTS

- Everytime you wash and dry your hands, use hand cream, especially if you live in a cold climate. Massage your nails and cuticles as well.
- A well-balanced diet is the cure for brittle or soft nails. Foods rich in calcium, vitamin A, and vitamin B will help build them up. Be sure your diet supplies sufficient amounts of protein and iron.
- If your cuticles are hard and in bad condition, soak them in warm olive or baby oil for a few minutes once a week to put them back in shape. Apply Vaseline to the cuticles overnight—it is an excellent restorative.
- Protect your nails (and hands) from dishwashing detergents and other harsh substances by wearing rubber gloves.
- Nails benefit from an occasional rest from nail polish.
- People react differently to different products. Try several brands of nail polish to see which ones stay longest and feel best on your hands.

HOW TO GIVE YOURSELF A PEDICURE

With a few added techniques to condition your feet, the basic manicure procedures will also give you "show-off" toes for summer sandals or slippers.

You will need:

A small pan or bowl large enough to soak your feet

Warm water with mild soap, bubble bath, or epsom salts (1 cup for each gallon of water)

Pumice stone

Nail scissors

Emery board
Cuticle cream
Orangewood stick
Nail polish, base coat, and sealer, if desired

1. Soak your feet for 10 minutes in a solution of warm water with soap, bubble bath, or epsom salts.

2. Remove your feet and use the pumice stone to gently rub off any rough or hardened skin from the heels, sides, and soles.

3. Dry your feet thoroughly.

4. Cut your nails along the edge, following the shape of the toe. Take care not to cut them too short or cut into the corners. Smooth off sharp nail edges with the coarse side of an emery board.

5. Rub in cuticle cream, massaging it in well. Push back the cuticles with the cotton-wrapped blunt end of an orangewood stick.

6. Apply hand cream to your feet, rubbing it in well. Knead and massage the sole, heel, and top of your foot.

7. For polishing, follow the manicure instructions from step 7 through step 14.

Attentively caring for your skin and your body is evidence of the new approach you are taking this week. You will find that the better you treat yourself, the better you will like yourself. And that is an important link to the positive attitude that will keep you sticking to your exercise and food plan as well.

After all, don't you think that your radiant skin and those soft graceful hands and feet deserve a slim, handsome body?

Marvelous Massage

Of all the rejuvenating treatments you can offer to your body, none is more magical than massage.

Massage is a marvelous therapeutic tool that gives you an unmatched feeling of well-being through touch. Long before man learned the secrets of medicine, he instinctively recognized the healing power of touch. The ancient Chinese and the Greeks and Romans all practiced the art of body manipulation as cures for various diseases.

Swedish massage, as practiced at Palm-Aire, also uses manipulation along established principles of anatomy and physiology. It is a system of active and passive exercises that affect the nervous and muscular systems and the general circulation. Massage alone will not make you lose weight, but Swedish massage does increase the natural interchange between the blood and tissue cells. This stimulates the metabolism, which regulates how the body burns calories. In combination with proper nutrition and exercise, it will aid a weight-reduction program.

Massage will also help soothe and refresh muscles that are stiff and tired from exercise, combating the aching feeling that might discourage you from your exercise regimen.

In today's stressful world, however, one of the principal functions of massage is simply to furnish unparalleled relaxation and comfort, to the spirit as well as the body. It has been proven that affirming and pleasing the body makes for good health. The body reacts to what we say and do to it. The more we denigrate ourselves, the more we dislike ourselves, and the more overweight and unhealthy we become. If we treat the body kindly, it reacts accordingly. With a massage, you show respect and appreciation for your body, and it may respond on levels beyond the physical.

The total relaxation achieved with massage helps stimulate the intellect as well as the body. While your body is stroked and comforted, your mind is free to focus on complex matters that may have seemed impossible to deal with in a tense, high-stress environment.

If you can afford professional massage as part of your fitness program, you will benefit in all of these ways. If not, you can still enjoy some of these rewards by learning to massage the parts of the body you can reach yourself—your foot, your neck, shoulders, face, and jaw.

Or you and a partner can learn to give each other the deep pleasure and benefits of overall massage, enriching both your physical and emotional exchange.

The Swedish massage techniques used at Palm-Aire are designed to benefit each organ of the body. Here are some of the basic ways it affects the different systems of the body.

The Circulatory System. The body depends on a complex and amazing pumping system. Because the heart is the pumping machine that keeps this system going, Swedish massage strokes are directed toward this key organ, aiding the action of the blood flow back to the heart and easing its work load.

The Lymphatic or Immune System. The lymph system is the body's vital waste disposal network, helping filter and dispose of wastes and toxins the blood stream leaves behind. It is key in helping the body resist infection. Because lymph vessels are most abundant just beneath the skin, they respond well to the stimulation of massage, which includes kneading and friction on the skin.

The Nervous System. This is the network that gives sensations of both pleasure and warning pain. Massage stimulates the nervous system to produce an overall sense of well-being.

The Muscular System. Muscles respond most dramatically to massage because they receive most of their nourishing blood supply when they are moved. Increased circulation induced by massage feeds the muscles, and regular massage has actually been shown to increase their size. Massage also helps muscles become firmer and more elastic so they are less susceptible to injury.

To provide the different kinds of stimulation the body needs for its various systems, massage consists of three basic therapeutic movements. Practice each one before you attempt a full massage.

Petrissage is a kneading motion that stimulates and rejuvenates the muscle by picking it up off the bone. This is done with one or two hands, very much like kneading dough. Grip as much muscle as you can and softly squeeze it away from the bone; release and repeat.

Tapotement, a steady slapping or hacking movement, stimulates nerve response by contracting and relaxing muscles and bringing fresh blood to the massage site. There are four ways to perform this technique: with the sides of your hands, the tips of your fingers, your cupped palms, and your closed fists. Movements are short and quick.

Effleurage, or stroking, is a long, smooth, even movement that directs blood circulation toward the heart, and soothes and relieves muscle fatigue. It can be done with your palms, knuckles, fingertips, or the ball of your thumb.

These three techniques are the foundation of a competent home massage. Two others often used by professionals may be learned as you become more proficient.

Friction, a deep circular movement, is used around the joints and bones. It employs the thumb, fingertips or palms, to limber up joints, tendons, and muscles.

Vibration, a trembling movement of the tissues, is done with hands or fingers to stimulate nerve centers.

THE HOME MASSAGE

The essentials for a home massage are simple. You will need:
• A massage table. A professional table is the best surface to use for a massage because the narrow width and comfortable height allows the massager to reach all parts of the body comfortably. If you do not have one, improvise by padding a long table or using your bed.

131

- A sheet to lie on.
- Towels to cover parts of the body not being massaged.
- Almond, sunflower, coconut, mineral, or any natural unrefined oil. Remember, don't use anything on your skin that you would not also use inside your body.

These simple tips will help you do a more effective job:
- Wear loose clothing with elbow-length or shorter sleeves.
- Warm the oil in your hand before applying to the body.
- Always work long strokes toward the heart to aid the circulatory system.
- Use both hands. Start gently and work up gradually in force. Remember that a beneficial massage requires some effort, both to give and to receive. Do not be afraid to use pressure; it is necessary to facilitate movement beneath the skin.
- Ask the recipient how he or she is feeling, whether more or less pressure is desired. Encourage a sense of sharing, both verbal and nonverbal. Avoid unnecessary conversation; most of the recipient's energy should go simply into feeling.

Here are basic step-by-step instructions for giving massage.

1. Begin with the recipient lying face up, eyes closed, with all parts of the body covered except the area to be massaged.

2. Massage the body in the following sequence: right arm, left arm, left leg, right leg, chest, and abdomen. Have the recipient turn over and massage the back of the left leg, the back of the right leg and then the back.

STROKE PATTERNS

Use the following stroke patterns for each part of the body, repeating each one 3 times unless otherwise directed:

ARMS

Use effleurage long strokes from wrist to shoulder by holding the arm with one hand and stroking it with the other. Stroke the palm of the hand first with one thumb and then the other. Then knead the wrist and hand with circular movements until you feel them getting warm. In successive order, knead, with circular motions, the fingers, hands, wrists, and whole arm from wrist to shoulder. Follow with tapotement and conclude by repeating the long strokes.

FRONT OF LEGS

Knead the foot top and bottom in small circles, concentrating on the adrenal point in the center of the sole of the foot. Do not use oil on the foot. Next knead the leg and thigh. Use long strokes to cover the entire leg from ankle to hip. Follow with tapotement, then repeat stroking.

CHEST

Starting in the center of the chest, stroke with both hands, working out to the sides, back to the center, up to the neck, and then back down to the center. Next stroke small circles from the sides of the neck to the top of the shoulders, using firm pressure. Knead the back and sides of the neck and then use circular tapping on sides of the chest. Repeat the stroking, follow with tapotement over the bronchial area of the chest; then end with one last long effleurage stroke.

ABDOMEN

Before starting on abdomen, lay one hand on the head and the other on the abdomen to indicate you are about to begin. Stroke with deep, circular movements; then knead both sides of the abdomen. Concentrate on the area on the left side over the colon, following the kneading with vibrating fingertips. Stroke again and then use firm pressure to stretch the stomach and abdomen downward. Now stretch the stomach muscles outward, then inward, and finish with a final long stroking.

BACK OF LEGS

Begin with long strokes from the ankle to the thigh. Follow by kneading the sole of the foot with your knuckles, and continue circular kneading up the leg to the thigh and hip, picking up the muscles. Follow with tapotement of the leg and thigh and conclude by stroking the entire leg.

BACK

Smoothly stroke the whole back, all the way to the skull; then stretch the back muscles from the spine outward. Next, vibrate each vertebra, starting at the top until the neck is relaxed and continue down the spine to the coccyx. Stretch, knead, and pick up the muscles of the entire back; follow with a side-to-side stretching movement and then circular kneading of the lower back and hips. Apply pressure to stretch the back muscles inward; then pick up the muscles of the upper back. Effleurage the whole back, follow with tapotement, and end with a final effleurage.

For the best effects, a glass of water or a cup of calming herbal tea should follow a massage.

SELF-MASSAGE

If a full massage is not possible, you can still enjoy the relaxing feeling massage offers by giving yourself a "minimassage." The areas you can reach yourself—your feet, hands, face, neck, and chest—will benefit from the attention, and you'll feel wonderful. Here are the how-to's for the Palm-Aire "minimassage."

THE FOOT

Foot reflexology is an Oriental technique that has been recently rediscovered in the West. It operates on the principle that each of the foot muscles represents an organ of the body. A foot reflex chart, available in most health food stores, shows the points corresponding to the organs that can be stimulated by foot massage. Impulses are sent to these various organs, simulating some of the benefits of full massage. Unlike the rest of the body, foot massage requires friction; oil is never applied to the foot. Knead the foot in small circles, using petrissage and effleurage techniques.

THE HAND

Gently massage the palm, the fleshy area under the thumb, the back of the hand, the forearm, and each finger, pulling the fingers slightly at each joint. Because the hand is a very sensitive area, you will quickly feel where the massage is doing the most good.

THE FACE

Massage the jaw, face, temples, and forehead, using a small circular kneading motion. Always work downward, away from the brain. Work the sensitive areas under the brow and around the sinuses.

THE NECK AND CHEST

Work down the sides of the neck to relieve neck pain, particularly along the large lateral neck muscles. Take a deep breath and massage the sternum to release your chest and shoulders. Massaging the scalp is also a good relaxation technique for the neck.

If you practice massage strokes until you have learned to perform them well, you will have given yourself and your partner a lifetime gift of pleasure and relaxation.

134

Makeup Magic

All of us, even the many glamorous stars who come to Palm-Aire, have features we wish we could change. We might like our eyes set wider apart, our noses shorter, our cheekbones heightened, or our chins made smaller.

The secret the stars have learned is one that you can share: Play up your best features and minimize your worst with the magic of makeup. Given the time to practice and experiment, you too can learn some of these professional tricks and make many flattering changes in your appearance.

To begin, pull your hair away from your face with a headband or clips, look in the mirror and analyze what you see carefully and honestly. What are the features you would like to change for more ideal balance in your face? Are your eyes too close together or too far apart? Is your nose too broad at the bridge or the base? Are your lips the same thickness? Is your jaw too square?

There is a makeup trick to correct each of these common complaints. The basic principle is a simple one: Light colors make an area stand out, while dark shading makes them recede. By using a light highlight down the center of your nose and darker foundation on the sides, for example, you can make it appear narrower. Light highlighting can also fool the eye, creating other illusions, such as making the creases around your mouth or the circles beneath your eyes almost disappear.

Remember that mirror lighting is important for achieving the right effect when you put on makeup. Be sure that you are working in light as close as possible to the light in which you will be seen, for example, natural light during the day and electric light after dark. Some makeup mirrors come with adjustable settings that simulate these different kinds of light. Whether you use an incandescent lamp or sit in daylight, position yourself so the light shines directly on your face without casting shadows. A mirror surrounded by bulbs is ideal because it illuminates all sides evenly. If you do not have one, place a lamp level with your face on either side of the mirror.

Follow the instructions below, using these professional tips from the makeup experts at Palm-Aire. Practice them at home in front of your mirror.

HOW TO APPLY MAKEUP

You will need:
Moisturizer
Base foundation matching your skin tone
Foundation or contour creams, one to two shades darker than the foundation for shading, one shade lighter for minimizing.
Blusher in a tone complementary to the base foundation
Concealer stick matching the base foundation
Translucent powder
Eye shadows in colors to complement your eye color
Eyeliner
Eyebrow pencil
Sponge makeup applicators

1. Makeup always starts with a light application of moisturizer. If you are fortunate enough to have a clear, smooth, and even complexion, you can skip any further foundation and use only moisturizer as a base. Next, apply contour and concealer layers. Then a layer of foundation blends them for a smooth overall look.

2. Use a concealer stick in the same color as your foundation to conceal pimples or blemishes.

3. Use a deeper shade of contour cream under your cheekbones for a hollower look. Confine it to the side of your face; imagine a line drawn straight down from the corner of your eye and do not go beyond it.

4. Use a lighter shade of contour cream on top of your cheekbone to accentuate the bone.

5. Apply a lighter foundation color or use a concealer stick to minimize lines around your mouth or circles under your eyes. For eyes, cover only the bottom line of the dark circle; applying concealing foundation to the puffy part of the eye will only emphasize it.

6. To define your jaw line, feel for the bone and use a darker shade of foundation just below it. Lift a heavy jaw by applying darker shades of foundation from the base of the midjaw up to midear in a long triangle just above the weighty part.

7. To make your nose appear more narrow, use a lighter foundation down the center of your nose and a darker shade of foundation on the sides. Darken the tip of your nose to shorten it.

8. Most people need a thin layer of foundation to even out the complexion. Use a color as close as possible to your natural skin color, just one shade darker at most. When you shop, test the color on your face, not on the back of your hand. For contour shaping, use the same tone as the base but one to two shades darker or lighter.

To apply foundation, place dots on your nose, cheeks, and chin and then blend them smoothly to cover the whole face. To avoid a heavy, masklike look, use a damp sponge to spread the foundation. Apply the foundation to your neck also, but thin the color as you work down to the base of your neck.

9. Blusher can give your face a big lift. Pick a color that blends well with your basic foundation: The lighter your skin tone, the lighter the blusher should be. Look straight into the mirror and draw an imaginary line straight down from the iris of your eye—the place where color begins just on the outside of the center pupil. This marks the highest point on your cheekbone. Apply a dot of color there at the center of the bone; then add two more dots, working outward along the bone and blend them in well until only a soft glow remains. If your face is round, emphasize the diagonal slant of your cheekbones. If your face is long, apply blusher in a horizontal line to give the impression of width. Lightly brush blush over each brow and on the chin for an extra glow.

10. Line your eyelids, top and bottom. To make your eyes appear more wide, apply eyeliner most heavily from the middle of the eye to the outside corner. Connect the top and bottom corners with liner to elongate your eyes.

Color liner can also be used on the edge of the lid just inside the eye to define the shape of the eye. Small eyes appear larger when the inside lids are lined with a soft white pencil.

11. Use eye shadow on upper lids, blending it into the crease. Eye color stroked on with a wet cotton applicator looks brighter and stronger.

Experiment to see how eye makeup can change the appearance of your eyes. A deeply colored eye shadow above the crease over the eye makes eyes stand out and minimizes puffiness. A lighter color close to the lashes appears to open up the eye. Neutral colors, such as beiges, browns, and grays, highlight the natural color of the eyes.

If your eyes are deep-set, a darker color applied toward the outside of the brow line and angled up at the outer corners will give the effect of pulling the eyes apart. Bring eyes closer together by blending darker shadow across the inside halves of the upper lid. Lift droopy eyes with light color on the outer corners of the lid. Elongate round eyes by applying shadow at the outer corner and lining the entire inside of the upper lids but only the outside halves of the lower portion.

Don't be afraid to use eye shadow. Experiment with a variety of shades to see which does the most for you. Have fun with color. Try, for example, to accent what you are wearing with just a touch of the color on the outer corners of your eyes.

12. Apply eyebrow pencil lightly to delineate your brows. The brow should arch where eye shadow color begins, nearest the center of your eye.

13. Use lip liner to define the shape of your mouth. If one lip is out of proportion, correct the shape with liner and then fill in with lipstick. The liner color should be slightly deeper than the lip color. If you want to wear a bright red color, but it is not flattering, using frosted or glossy colors may allow you to get away with a brighter shade.

Lipstick and blusher colors should be in the same tones; you can actually use a touch of lip color to pick up and match your basic blush.

14. Set makeup with a light dusting of translucent powder.

15. Use restraint for a natural look in the daytime, and more blusher and richer lip color for glamour at night.

Investing time to learn to use makeup properly will return a lifetime of dividends. The more you know about makeup magic, the more adept you will become at hiding the flaws and putting your best face forward.

CROWNING GLORY

A flattering haircut is the crowning touch to an attractive face, and a skilled stylist is a woman's best friend.

But it's up to you to get the most from your hairstylist. Like makeup, your hairstyle should balance your face and compensate for your weak points. It should support your personal image, not simply mirror the fashion of the day, and in the busy world we live in, a haircut should be easy to maintain. As your face begins to show signs of age, your hair should be styled softly, to flatter and to divert the eye up and away from aging lines.

According to the stylists at Palm-Aire, women too often simply let a hairdresser make decisions for them without letting him or her know what they want. "Put your hairdresser up against the wall," one stylist jokes. "Ask her to justify your hairstyle according to your own face, age, and life-style. Beware of a stylist who specializes in the newest fad haircuts. Find a hairdresser who will look hard at who *you* are, not just automatically try to give you the latest look. When your hairdresser suggests a new haircut, ask *why* it's for you and what it will do for your face. Don't allow yourself to be put into a cookie-cutter mold."

Keeping your hair shiny and healthy is also important to its appearance. A hair conditioning treatment is part of your beauty routine this week, one that ought to be repeated regularly. Look for a protein pack or ask your hairdresser to suggest an appropriate, dependable product for you.

Here are more basic hair-care do's and don'ts:

- Use only natural-bristle hairbrushes, never nylon. Brush often with your head down for better circulation.
- Scalp massage stimulates circulation and helps keep hair healthy, and it's also quite relaxing. Use your fingertips and a circular kneading motion.
- Use protein packs to renew your hair if it has been damaged by the sun.
- If your hair is oily or dry, use the proper shampoo for your hair type.
- Always use a mild shampoo, not one containing a harsh detergent. Read the labels carefully.

- Remember that you are cleaning your scalp as well as your hair; take a few minutes to massage shampoo into your scalp.
- A vinegar rinse restores the perfect pH to oily hair.
- Unless your hair is very dry, wash it daily; one shampoo and rinse is sufficient.
- Always rinse thoroughly—and then rinse again. Shampoo residues dry the scalp.
- Conditioners after shampooing keep hair smooth and manageable.
- Dry your hair gently; keep the temperature warm rather than hot, and never hold a blow dryer too close to your head.
- Even if you prefer coloring your hair at home, you would be wise to discuss color with a professional before you make a decision regarding which shade and what type of coloring to use.

Back Talk

"Oh, My Aching Back" is a complaint we hear often at Palm-Aire and one that undermines the best intentions. It's hard to be at your best or stay with an exercise plan when you're feeling the discomfort of a bad back.

Back ailments can hit anyone. They strike 80 percent of all men sometime during their lives, and are on the increase for women as well. Traditionally, women remained limber because they did more bending and stretching in household chores and child care, but as more and more women join the work force, they are sharing the back pain that a desk job and lack of exercise can bring.

But while back problems are common, they are also preventable. Men and women alike can learn to stop backaches before they start. Here is the know-how that Palm-Aire's specialists pass along to guests.

Improving your posture is the single most important thing you can do for your back. Good posture prevents strain, not only on the back, but on muscles, joints, ligaments, and internal organs. Posture is more than a matter of "standing tall."

It should be considered in all activities: sitting, resting, working, playing, and exercising—not just standing.

The second crucial step in strengthening the back is to make the abdominal muscles that support it stronger; this is an area where women are often weak.

A good preventive program of stretching exercises can stop back problems before they start. The areas that are most important are the upper legs, particularly the hamstring muscles at the back of the leg, and the buttocks, lower back, and stomach.

Learning to avoid movements and positions that strain the back is another wise preventive measure. Here are the Palm-Aire Spa exercise experts' hints to protect the back and exercises to strengthen it. If you learn to live with them, even a weak back can gradually return to being a comfortable, functional part of you. Prevention is the best cure. If you've got a bad back, 15 minutes of daily exercise can keep you pain-free!

BACK RULES TO LIVE BY

- Always sit all the way back in a chair with your back erect. At your desk, put your feet on a small footstool or a large reference book about 9 inches thick to take pressure off your lower back.
- Sleep on a firm mattress; if your mattress is not firm, put a ¾-inch-thick plywood board underneath it.
- If you sleep on your back, keep a pillow under your knees, not under your head. Keep your knees bent when you sleep on your side. Do not sleep on your stomach.
- When driving a car, keep the seat forward so your body is erect. On long trips, stop every hour or so and walk around to relieve tension and relax your muscles.
- When doing any work that requires standing for a long period of time, place one foot on a stool or bench to ease the strain.
- Be conscious of your posture and avoid swayback. Tuck your pelvis forward to straighten your back.
- Get regular exercise and make a conscious effort to relax several times a day.
- If your back acts up, see your doctor at once—do not wait for it to become worse.

Exercises for Better Back Care

GENERAL INSTRUCTIONS:

Follow your doctor's instructions carefully. Start slowly and gradually increase speed and repetition. Don't overdo it. Exercise on a rug or mat. Put a pillow under your neck. Dress comfortably—no shoes or socks. Stop doing any exercise that causes pain until you have checked with your doctor.

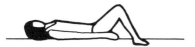

• Lie on your back with your knees bent and your feet flat on the floor. Take a deep breath and relax. Press the small of your back against the floor and tighten your stomach and buttocks muscles. This should cause the lower end of the pelvis to rotate forward. Hold for 5 seconds. Relax. Repeat 10 times.

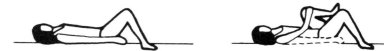

• Lie on your back with your knees bent and your feet flat on the floor. Take a deep breath and relax. Grasp one knee with both hands and pull it as close to your chest as possible. Return to the starting position. Straighten your legs. Return to the starting position. Repeat 10 times for each leg, alternating your legs.

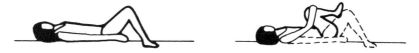

• Lie on your back with your knees bent and your feet flat on the floor. Take a deep breath and relax. Grasp both knees and pull them as close to your chest as possible. Return to the starting position. Straighten your legs. Return to the starting position. Relax. Repeat 10 times.

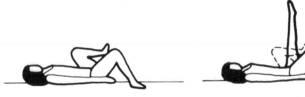

• Lie on your back with your knees bent and your feet flat on the floor. Take a deep breath and relax. Draw one knee to your chest. Then point that leg upward as far as possible. Return to the starting position. Relax. Repeat 10 times, alternating your legs. (*Note:* This exercise is not recommended for patients with sciatic pain.)

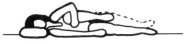

• Lie on your side with your knees bent. Take a deep breath and relax. Slide your uppermost knee toward your chest as far as possible. Return to the starting position. Relax. Repeat 10 times on each side.

• Lie on your stomach with your head on your hands. Take a deep breath and relax. Tighten your buttocks muscles and hold for 2 seconds. Relax. Repeat 10 times.

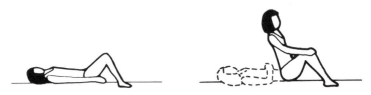

• (*Note:* This exercise should not be started until the others have been done for several weeks.) Lie on your back with your knees bent and your feet flat on the floor. Take a deep breath and relax. Pull up to a sitting position while keeping your knees bent. Return to the starting position. Relax. Repeat 10 times. (*Note:* Having someone hold your feet down can facilitate this exercise.)

144

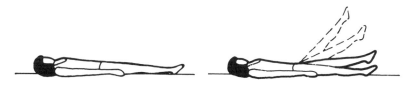

• Lie on your back with your legs straight out and your arms at your sides. Take a deep breath and relax. Raise your legs one at a time as high as is comfortable and then lower to the floor as slowly as possible. Repeat 5 times for each leg.

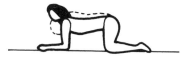

• Get down on your hands and knees. Take a deep breath and relax. Pull your stomach in and curve your back upward. Let your head hang down. Now arch your back and look up; then relax. Repeat 10 times.

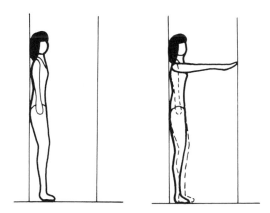

• Stand with your back against a doorframe. Place your heels 4 inches away from the frame. Take a deep breath and relax. Press the small of your back against the doorframe. Tighten your stomach and buttocks muscles, allowing your knees to bend slightly. This should cause the lower end of the pelvis to rotate forward (as in the first exercise, above). Press your neck up against the doorframe. Press both hands against the opposite side of the frame and straighten both knees. Hold for 2 seconds. Relax. Repeat 10 times.

BACK-CARE PROGRAM

This guide is designed to help you begin to correct the positions and movements that may aggravate your back problem. Particular emphasis is placed on rest positions, because even in these positions it is possible to strain your neck and back. Practicing good posture in all your activities is another important step toward a stronger, healthier back.

DO

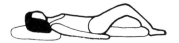

BACK-LYING

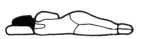

SIDE-LYING
Curl up on side with knees bent.
Optional—pillow between knees.

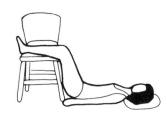

ALTERNATE REST POSITION

DON'T

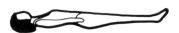

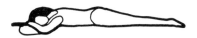

Above positions cause swayback

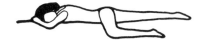

DO

UP AND DOWN FROM BED

DOWN

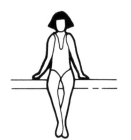

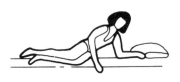

1. Sit on edge of bed.
2. Bring both arms to one side.
3. Lower side of body to bed keeping knees bent 45°.
4. Put feet into bed.
5. Remain on side or roll to back.

UP

1. Roll to side.
2. Push with hands to sitting position.
3. Keep knees bent and swing legs over edge of bed.

DO   DON'T

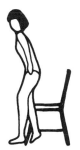

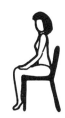

SITTING

Good body mechanics when sitting down in a chair.
If a chair is too high, swayback is increased.
Knees higher than hips flattens the
  lower back, legs straight on ottoman
  strains the lower back.

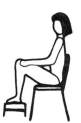

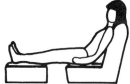

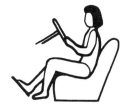

CAR

Car seat closer to steering wheel
flattens the lower back.

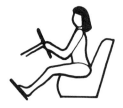

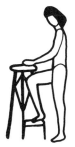

STANDING

A footrest will relieve the swayback
and help to flatten the back.

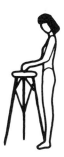

147

DO   DON'T

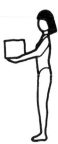 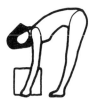

Bend at the hips and knees and not at the waist.
Hold and carry objects close to you.

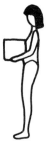 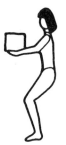

Keep back rounded as you return to standing from
squat.

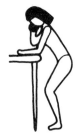 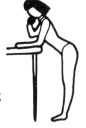

Never bend over without bending knees and tucking
buttocks under.

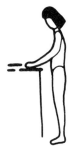 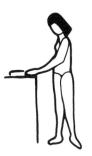

Always face your work and turn by pivoting your
feet first.

DO   DON'T

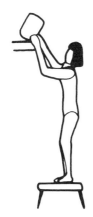 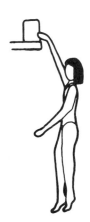

Keep buttocks tucked under as you reach. Use a
stool and avoid unnecessary reaching.

MORE RULES

- Avoid bending from the waist only; bend your hips and knees.
- Avoid lifting heavy objects higher than your waist.
- Always turn and face the object you wish to lift.
- Avoid carrying unbalanced loads.
- Hold heavy objects close to your body.
- Never carry or move anything that you cannot handle with ease.
- Avoid sudden movements. Learn to move more deliberately.
- Change positions frequently.
- When mopping, vacuuming, raking, hoeing, etc., always work with the tool close to your body. Never use a "giant" step and a long reach in these activities.
- Sit down to dress and put on socks and shoes. Don't bend from the waist while trying to balance on one foot.
- Women should wear low heels.
- Avoid exercise and activities that arch or strain your lower back (for example, backward bends or forward bends to touch toes).
- When you cough or sneeze, round your back and bend your knees slightly.
- When making a bed, do so from a kneeling position.

149

Heart to Heart

The Palm-Aire Plan, the new healthful menus, and the more active, low-stress life-style it teaches you can do something far more important for you than slim your waistline. It may save your life.

Every year about a million Americans have heart attacks, and more than half of them die. Most of these victims had not even known that they had heart disease until it was too late.

We can't predict who is going to suffer a heart attack, or when, but we can pick out certain "risk factors" that characterize a likely heart attack candidate. At Palm-Aire, guests are given a cardiac risk evaluation developed by the New York State Education Department to help people measure and understand their own risk. Try it and see how you measure up.

If your risk is moderate or above, it's time to pay serious attention and see if you can lower your score in the next 6 months.

Some primary risk factors, such as your age, sex, and family history, cannot be changed. Those you *can* change are high blood pressure, abnormally high cholesterol levels, obesity, physical in-activity, high stress, and cigarette smoking.

High blood pressure, once detected, can be corrected by medication. Mildly high pressure may be lowered naturally simply by exercising, cutting down on sodium and caffeine, and losing weight and keeping it off. The key is to have your blood pressure tested—NOW—so your physician can counsel you and prescribe what is needed.

Research has shown that cholesterol levels will go down if you reduce the amount of animal fat in your diet *and* increase exercise. It's the combination that makes the difference. With the Palm-Aire Plan, you are beginning both a healthier diet and a more active life-style, and your body will soon reflect these changes.

Regular aerobic exercise alone has been shown to help the heart in many ways. The increased circulation and rate of metabolism caused by exercise strengthens the heart. To meet the body's increased demands during regular exercise, the heart develops more and larger blood vessels and muscles that can contract more easily, changes that also make it better able to cope with challenges, such as the insufficient oxygen flow that occurs during a heart attack. Improved blood clotting mechanisms, lowered blood and body fat profiles, lowered blood pressure, and reduced tension levels are other benefits from aerobics.

Furthermore, even a moderate amount of exercise can extend your life significantly. A recent study of 17,000 Harvard alumni found that those who did any combination of walking, climbing stairs, sports, and exercise that used 2,000 calories or more a week had death rates one-quarter to one-third less than nonexercisers of the same age. A brisk, 3-mile daily walk is enough to burn up to 2,000 calories, and this is something even the busiest of us can fit into our routines, simply by walking all or part way to some of our destinations.

Another Harvard study found that a stronger heart was not the only benefit of regular exercise. Active women were shown to be less likely than sedentary women to develop breast cancer, perhaps because they have a smaller percentage of fat in their bodies. Fatty tissue releases cancer-promoting estrogen into the bloodstream. Exercise also has been shown to help ward off adult-onset diabetes, strokes, osteoporosis, and depression. And it helps delay aging by slowing the decline in certain body functions, such as reaction time and responses to visual stimuli.

The Palm-Aire Plan will motivate you to change your diet and get your body into action, but there are still other important health risk factors you can control. Of all the changes you can make that will affect your longevity and good health, giving up smoking heads the list. We all know that smoking has been implicated as a cause of cancer.

Statistical evidence has proven that smoking hurts the arteries. Nicotine in the smoke causes the blood vessels to become constricted and, at the same time, elevates the heart rate, creating a dramatic increase in blood pressure. There is pressure on the arteries to accommodate additional flow through smaller spaces.

Smoke inhaled into the lungs also diffuses into the blood as carbon monoxide, reducing the oxygen-carrying capacity of the blood and forcing the heart to work harder to provide the same amount of oxygen.

There are at least two more good reasons to give up smoking. One is the improved breathing capacity that will make your exercising much easier. The second is pure and simple vanity. Because it affects the circulation, smoking dulls the healthy good looks of your skin. Simply stated, you will look better and feel better if you stop smoking.

Psychological stress has been shown to have some of the same adverse physical affects as smoking. Stress also results in constriction of the blood vessels, elevating blood pressure. Blood analysis has shown that blood cholesterol levels also are elevated in times of stress.

We hear a lot of people say, "I can't change my job or my life-style, so what can I do about stress?"

Regular aerobic exercise is one proven stress reliever. But there are many other ways to relieve stress in your life—and possibly even change your life. Let's take a look at some of them in the next chapter.

PALM-AIRE CARDIAC RISK PROFILE

Age	10–20 Years	I	21–30 Years	2	31–40 Years	3
Heredity:Parents, and Siblings	No family history of CVD	I	One with CVD over 60 years	2	Two with CVD over 60 years	3
Weight	More than 5 lbs. below standard weight	O	– 5 to – 15 lbs. of standard weight	I	5–20 lbs. overweight	2
Tobacco Smoking	Nonuser	O	Occasional cigar or pipe	I	Cigarettes 10 or less/day	2
Exercise	Intensive job and recreational exertion	O	Moderate job and recreational exertion	I	Sedentary job and intensive recreation	2
Cholesterol*	Below 180 mg %	I	181–205 mg %	2	206–230 mg %	3
Systolic Blood Pressure*	Below 110 mm Hg	O	111–130 mm Hg	I	131–140 mm Hg	2
Diastolic Blood Pressure*	Below 80 mm Hg	O	80–85 mm Hg	I	86–90 mm Hg	2
Gender	Female	I	Female over 45 years	2	Male	4
Resting EKG*	Normal	O	Borderline	2	Frequent PVC's	3
Stress	No stress	I	Occasional mild stress	2	Frequent mild stress	3
Present CVD Symptoms	None	O	Occasional fast pulse and/or irregular rhythm	2	Frequent fast pulse and/or irregular rhythm	4
Past Personal History CVD	Completely benign	O	CVD Symptoms Not confirmed by physician	2	History of CVD Symptoms examined by physician	4
Diabetes	No symptoms Negative family history	O	Latent Positive family history	I	Chemical	3
Gout	No symptoms Negative family history	O	Family history	I	Elevated uric acid (8 mg % +) No Symptoms	2

6–14 = Risk well below average   26–32 = Risk moderate

15–19 = Risk below average   33–40 = Risk dangerous; you must reduce your score

20–25 = Risk generally average

			Initial score	Six months later
41–50 Years **4**	51–60 Years **6**	60 + Years **8**		
One death from CVD under 60 years **4**	Two deaths from CVD under 60 years **6**	Three deaths from CVD under 60 years **7**		
21–35 lbs. overweight **3**	36–50 lbs. overweight **5**	51–65 lbs. overweight **7**		
Cigarettes 11–20 per day **4**	Cigarettes 21–30 per day **6**	Cigarettes over 31 per day **10**		
Sedentary job and moderate recreation **4**	Sedentary job and light recreation **6**	Sedentary job No special exercise **8**		
231–255 mg % **4**	256–280 mg % **5**	281–300 mg % **7**		
141–160 mm Hg **3**	161–180 mm Hg **5**	Above 180 mm Hg **7**		
91–95 mm Hg **4**	96–100 mm Hg **7**	101 and above **9**		
Bald male **5**	Bald, short male **6**	Bald, short, stocky male **7**		
Conduction defect **4**	Ischemia **7**	Infarction **10**		
Frequent moderate stress **4**	Frequent high stress **5**	Constant high stress **7**		
Dizziness on exertion **6**	Occasional angina **8**	Frequent angina **10**		
Mild CVD No present treatment **6**	CVD Under treatment **8**	Hospitalized for CVD **10**		
Mild dietary control **5**	Moderate Oral Rx control **7**	Severe Insulin control **9**		
New onset Gout early detected **3**	Repeated chronic gouty attacks **5**	Gout with renal and osteo complications **8**		
		Total		

Check Total Score Evaluation for Precautions and/or Limitations

Source: Courtesy of the New York State Education Department.
*To be determined by a physician.

Stress and De-stress

Most guests come to the Palm-Aire Spa hoping for more than weight loss. They are also looking for an oasis of calm, a chance to de-stress from their busy, hectic lives.

While a week off cannot always solve life's problems, it can provide an opportunity to learn how to cope better with the stresses of everyday living. Equally important, it can also offer an opportunity to consider ways of improving the quality of that daily life.

This same kind of awareness is a gift you can give yourself during your Palm-Aire Plan week at home. You can learn de-stressing techniques. You can also set aside special time for reevaluation, time to take a good hard look at what you can do in the weeks ahead to make your life a lot less harried and a lot more rewarding. Simply making time to take stock of yourself, and your present responses to life's tensions, is a very healthy start.

Remember that stress in itself is not a bad thing. Any change in life causes stress, even the good changes. A popular stress measure chart devised a number of years ago by Doctors Thomas Holmes and Richard Rahe rated marriage and reconciliation high on the stress list, and a promotion at work more stressful than having difficulties with in-laws.

Some stress also comes with any unfamiliar situation: going to a party where you don't know many people, going to a new city or country, even visiting a spa for the first time. Stress accompanies any challenge, whether it is doing our jobs or measuring up in sports. We need some amount of stress to mobilize energy and motivate us to perform well. Too much safety can leave you feeling bored and unfulfilled.

Stress becomes *dis*tress only when an overload leaves you tense and agitated, not feeling or behaving at your best. Instead of motivating, too much stress does the opposite: It saps energy and undermines good intentions, including a resolve to watch your weight. For some people, compulsive eating is often a reaction to tension.

The solution is to learn to head off stress overload before it does damage to our bodies and spirits.

The Palm-Aire stress-reduction workshops begin by helping you look at what kinds of situations you perceive as stressful and how your body reacts to them. Besides the personal stresses in our lives, many unavoidable outside sources of distress surround us every day. There are environmental stresses like weather, noise, traffic, and time pressures. Our bodies react stressfully to biological changes, too, like aging, accidents, illness, a poor diet, or lack of sleep. Examining the ways you respond to different types of stress allows you to learn how to better control these responses.

Palm-Aire guests go over the following checklist to identify the common signs of distress. Which of these symptoms have you experienced?

MOOD & DISPOSITION SIGNS
..... *I become overexcited.*
..... *I worry.*
..... *I feel insecure.*
..... *I have difficulty sleeping at night.*
..... *I become easily confused and forgetful.*
..... *I become uncomfortable and ill at ease.*
..... *I become nervous.*

VISCERAL SIGNS
..... *My stomach becomes upset.*
..... *I feel my heart pounding.*
..... *I sweat profusely.*
..... *My hands become moist.*

..... *I feel light-headed or faint.*
..... *I experience "cold chills."*
..... *My face becomes flushed and hot.*

MUSCULOSKELETAL SIGNS
..... *My fingers and hands shake.*
..... *I can't sit or stand still.*
..... *I develop twitches.*
..... *My head begins to ache.*
..... *I feel my muscles become tense or stiff.*
..... *I stutter or stammer when I speak.*
..... *My neck becomes stiff.*

Most of these common reactions boil down to the "fight-or-flight" response that had been part of man's makeup ever since the day the cave man mustered courage to brave the hunt for food. The same survival instincts that come into play when we are faced with physical danger occur when the psychological perils of the modern world attack us. They break down into two categories:

FIGHT *(increases these responses)*	FLIGHT *(slows these responses)*
muscle tension	*blood to extremities*
heart rate	*digestion*
respiration	*saliva glands*
adrenalin	*(common effects of these*
sweat glands	*slow-downs are dry mouth, cold*
energy mobilization	*hands and feet, involuntary*
hearing acuity	*urination or diarrhea)*
long vision	

As you can see, many of these "fight" responses can be positive—unless they get out of hand. When stress becomes chronic, the symptoms become more intense until they eventually interfere with our ability to function well. Too much psychological stress can actually produce physical responses—high blood pressure, headaches, or asthma—that require medical attention.

Ideally, we hope to intervene before stress escalates beyond what we can handle. Feeling in control of circumstances that affect us is the key to beating stress. Feeling helpless magnifies stress. Once you decide to take more responsibility for your own well-being, you can learn ways to gain more control, whether that means temporary relief or a permanent life-style change.

Wanting to be in control is almost a reflex reaction. Take a simple situation such as standing in line at the bank. Suppose it is lunchtime and you are going to get back to work late because the line is not moving. You have little power over the line, but the natural instinct is to gain whatever control you can muster. The first response may be simply to shift from foot to foot, a small way of exercising control over the body to ease tenseness. Next might come a little pep talk to psych yourself into being calmer, telling the mind to relax. Eventually there is a compulsion for action of some kind, perhaps moving into a different line just to create some kind of movement. The final response often is to assert yourself out loud, either by complaining to the next person in line or, perhaps more constructively, by looking for the manager.

These are almost automatic responses. There are other more deliberate techniques that you can employ to help control responses to stress. They fall into four categories.

FOUR RESPONSES TO STRESS

SOCIAL ENGINEERING

Social engineering simply means doing what we can to limit the amount of stress we must encounter. When circumstances permit, *avoidance* is one of the easiest of these techniques. One example of avoidance would be to stay away from known stress producers, such as going to the bank at lunch hour, perhaps by finding another bank with an automatic teller or more convenient hours. If you know that traffic jams or crowded subways or buses raise your stress level, you might try to avoid them and allow enough time to walk at least part of the way to your job, getting in some aerobic exercise and burning off calories as well as steam. Think about your routines and see how many of life's petty annoyances you might be able to drop by some crafty avoidance.

When it comes to major life decisions, if you understand that changes produce stress, you can sometimes control overload by avoiding too many major changes at once. If you are in a new marriage, for example, it's not the best time to look for a new job. If you have just had a traumatic separation, such as a death or divorce, it may be wise to wait a while before moving to a new home.

Time management is another social engineering technique that can ben-

160

efit many busy people. There are whole books and many courses designed to help you organize and make better use of your time, but the gist of their message is simply to think through your priorities and focus your energy on one thing at a time. That way you will have the satisfaction of making progress on the most important tasks each day, rather than scattering your efforts and feeling frustrated and stressed because nothing is accomplished.

One of the most familiar examples of time-management suggests how to control the overflow of paperwork that clutters many offices and homes. It directs you to divide papers into A, B, and C categories. The A's get immediate attention, the B's get reviewed only when the A's are finished, and the least important C's may either go into a drawer for perusal at a later, idle time or into the wastebasket! You can give your daily activities A, B, and C ratings as well, and stop cluttering your time with the unimportant ones to make more time for what really matters.

Another revealing exercise that may help you reorganize your time is to make a list of all the activities that presently fill your life. Divide them into categories, such as socializing, work, parenting, sports, exercise, hobbies, television, reading, cooking, housework, meetings, shopping, eating, and the like. Now draw a circle, and divide it into different-sized pie-shaped sections representing the activities that fill your normal week and the amount of time you spend doing them. Fill in everything you do except for sleep.

It is often a surprise to see your time patterns laid out so graphically. If you see that you are putting a disproportionate amount of time and energy into categories that are not really productive, continue with the second part of this exercise. Draw another circle and set up an ideal time pattern. Now think about what it would take to change reality to make it closer to your ideal. A new assistant? A smaller home? Resigning from a few activities? Less commuting time? Less time on the phone? A new job? A loan?

You may begin to see that impossible dreams are not quite as impossible as they seemed. Believing that you have no control and no choices in your life contributes to stress. With creativity, and the will to make changes, there may be choices you have not considered that can make your life more rewarding.

Goal setting is a somewhat similar idea. One common problem in today's world is that we simply have too many options. When stress begins to close in, it may be time to examine your life-style and modify your goals a bit—to stop trying to be and do too many things at once. Thinking about what you really want out of life and writing down the goals most important to you make it easier to eliminate projects that overload your schedule but do not help you reach your goals. Set aside a specific time this week—perhaps while you are soaking in the tub or when you have completed a relaxation exercise—to take a good hard look at your present life and identify some constructive changes you can record as future goals in the charts at the end of this book. Think about which phases of your life cause the stressful responses you checked off at the beginning of this chapter and how many of them you might be able to eliminate.

One way to approach goal-setting is to fantasize a bit about what your life would be like if it could be anything you chose, no limit on your time, finances, looks, or talent. Close your eyes and forget about reality. Pretend it is 5 years from today. Where are you? What are your surroundings like? What is the weather like? How do you look and dress? It's 5 years from now, remember. Who are you with? If you have children, what do they look like? Go over your day, hour by hour, from the time you wake up until you go to bed. This is your ideal day, so there are no limitations. What is the nature of your work or activity? Are you busy or relaxed, working alone or with others, indoors or out? What kind of work are you doing? What happens at the end of the day? How about later on in the evening?

No one is going to know about this particular fantasy but you, no censors, no pragmatists allowed, so dream away. How do others acknowledge you? How much money do you have? What kind of excitement, stimulation, and learning are you experiencing? What kind of challenges are you facing? What are your leisure activities? At what do you excel?

Now consider all the possible steps you could take to begin moving a little closer to your ideal—not to attain it, necessarily, but to make progress toward it. How can you rewrite your life script?

Here's another variation on the theme. Make a list of all the things you'd like to do before you die, long and short term. Maybe you want to go to China or learn to paint or speak a foreign language or go back to school. Maybe you have an entirely different set of goals. Perhaps you want to lose 20 pounds and have a facelift.

Whatever you really want, think about how many of these things you might accomplish within the next year if you really wanted to badly enough. What about in the next 5 years—or 10? What would it take to do it?

All of this fantasizing is more than just wishful thinking. The extent to which your dreams remain fantasies may be up to you. Limiting beliefs keep many of us from reaching our goals. While some goals may be unattainable, if you decide what you want and make up your mind to go after it with all the energy and determination you can muster, you can probably go a long way toward making some of your dreams come true—or at least come close enough to make for a very meaningful improvement in your life.

PERSONALITY AND ATTITUDE ADJUSTMENT

Goal-setting overlaps somewhat into the second category of stress-control techniques, which deal more with attitude than actions. A more positive outlook makes many unavoidable stresses seem less significant in the overall scheme of things. Anything that helps you gain that more positive outlook belongs in this group of techniques—from psychotherapy to assertiveness training to support groups to reading appropriate books or articles—and gives you more insight into yourself.

It is hard to view life positively when you don't feel well. Eating a well-balanced diet and getting enough sleep and exercise are not just matters of vanity. Being emotionally fit is as vital as being physically fit, and remembering this may help you stick to your exercise and diet resolves.

If you are fighting to end long-established harmful habits, find a support group of people with the same problems and goals; it can make the difference between success and failure. Probably, the most familiar and most successful self-help group is Alcoholics Anonymous. Today, there are also support groups for those who want to lose weight, stop smoking, break a drug dependency, and conquer many other kinds of habits.

Support means even more in periods when life's crises bring us down. The opportunity to share feelings with others who are experiencing similar problems can do much to make stressful times easier to bear. Support groups are available for those undergoing divorce or serious illness, as well as for people facing single parenthood or the urgent need to find a new job. Joining one of these groups can help you change your perspective and find hope during difficult moments.

Whatever the cause of stress, humor is one guaranteed antidote. Palm-Aire Spa guests are reminded that laughter actually produces endorphins, which act as a natural pain killer in the body. Look for the funny side of things, take a less serious, more playful attitude toward life and make time for simple fun and laughter—it may do more to combat stress than any other single technique.

One Palm-Aire counselor recommends collecting a humor scrapbook full of cartoons and clippings you find funny. It keeps you on the lookout for life's lighter side.

FITNESS ACTIVITIES

The "Fight-or-Flight" syndrome, the increased adrenaline and respiration, which is switched on by stress, is actually the body's way of getting ready for action. While we no longer have to fight off physically most of the threats to our well-being, we can still let the body work off its tension very efficiently by allowing it to move into action with exercise. The active workouts of aerobics are proven stress reducers—but only when they are noncompetitive activities. If you strain to compete in a race or even push yourself to meet a speed or distance goal you have set, the exercise will only produce its own kind of tension.

RELAXATION TRAINING

The most immediate way to ease stress is to learn how to help the body turn off its responses temporarily with specific relaxation techniques. In order for relaxation techniques to work when you need them, you must practice and become adept at doing them. Here are seven ways to relax for you to try, one each day, as part of the Palm-Aire Plan. See which ones work best for you, and keep practicing those you prefer daily for about 2 weeks until they become second nature. When your body is conditioned to relax in this way, you will find, after a while, that you will begin to relax a bit just thinking about the exercise. If you use background music, hearing it will also begin to make you relax.

DEEP BREATHING. Breathing deeply and slowly can help reduce anxiety, depression, and fatigue. (It comes first because it is not only a valuable technique on its own but part of other relaxation exercises.) The aim is to learn to breathe from the diaphragm rather than from the chest, and it's done simply by expanding the abdomen as you inhale and contracting it as you exhale. The longer you practice deep breathing, the more effective it becomes.

1. Lie down with your knees bent, feet on the floor about 8 inches apart.

2. Place one hand on your abdomen and one on your chest. Inhale slowly and deeply through your nose into your abdomen. Feel your abdomen rise with your hand. Your chest should move only slightly and only when the abdomen moves.

3. Exhale through your mouth with a gentle whooshing sound, pulling in your abdomen and drawing it back toward your spine.

4. Continue for 5 to 10 minutes, inhaling for 5 seconds and exhaling for 10 seconds. Notice the lessening of tension when you have completed this exercise.

164

"PALMING." Resting the eyes is an important way of reestablishing balance and reducing unnecessary stress. This exercise relaxes not just your eyes but your whole body, and you can do it anywhere—from your office to a seat on a train or plane.

1. Sit or lie down and take a few moments to breathe deeply.

2. Now gently close your eyes and place the palms of your hands over your eyes, with your fingers crossing over your forehead.

3. Use memory and imagination to create a perfect field of black. See it so *black* that you cannot recall anything darker. Do not try to produce any experience. Simply *allow* the darkness to happen. Continue for 2 to 3 minutes, breathing easily.

4. Remove your hands and open your eyes slowly.

You can repeat this exercise several times a day, whenever you need to relax. It can also leave you ready for a wonderful relaxed night's sleep.

PROGRESSIVE RELAXATION. Many people have no idea that some of their muscles are chronically tense. This exercise works on the principle of opposites. It first tenses muscles to their utmost in order to relax them totally.

1. Get into a comfortable position, either lying down or sitting in a chair with a back high enough to support your head.

2. Clench your hands and arms as tight as you can, making fists and bulging biceps, and hold for 5 to 7 seconds. Now let go all at once and let your muscles relax completely for 30 seconds.

3. Follow the same procedure for your head, face, throat, and shoulders. Hunch your shoulders high, and concentrate especially on your face muscles by wrinkling your forehead as tight as you can, squinting your eyes, tensing your jaw, pursing your lips, and pushing your tongue to the roof of your mouth. After 5 to 7 seconds, relax completely.

4. Now repeat for your chest, stomach, and lower back, concentrating separately on each part of your body.

5. Repeat for your thighs, buttocks, calves, and feet.

6. As you relax, say to yourself, "The tension is going away. I am feeling relaxed. I am letting go more and more." Breathe more deeply. With practice, you will find that by telling them to, the muscles actually will begin to relax more and more.

RELAXING WITH MUSIC. Here is an exercise that will calm you, energize you, and make you ready to face the rest of the day with renewed energy. (Suggestions for relaxing music are found at the end of this chapter.)

1. Turn on relaxing orchestral music—no words, just music.

2. Sit comfortably and quietly or lie down on the floor.

3. Tell yourself that you are going to use the next 15 minutes to rebalance, to heal, to relax yourself.

4. Surrender the weight of your body, allowing the chair or floor to support you.

5. Close your eyes, gently cutting out visual stimulation and distraction.

6. As you inhale, repeat to yourself "I am . . ."

7. As you exhale, say ". . . relaxed."

8. Continue to breathe normally, not trying to change your reactions in any way. Just continue to repeat: "I am" with inhalation, "relaxed" with exhalation, and feel it happening.

9. As your mind begins to wander, gently bring it back to the awareness of breath and your statement, "I am relaxed."

10. Allow the music to soothe you and bring you into a deeper state of relaxation.

11. To conclude, slowly stretch your hands and feet, your arms and legs, your whole body.

12. Now open your eyes a sliver at a time.

A CANDLE MEDITATION. This exercise can help to clear your mind when pressures pile up. The purpose is to learn to visualize one thing at a time with your full awareness. It takes practice to screen out the distractions your mind will raise, but once mastered, this technique helps keep you more centered and calm.

1. Light a candle in a semidarkened room and place it about 18 inches from where you will be sitting, at your eye level.

2. Sit down in a comfortable chair and look at the candle. Become absorbed with it.

3. As thoughts arise, keep pushing them back and bringing your attention

back to the candle and flame. Try not to analyze or describe what is taking place. Simply let it happen, *be* with it.

4. Close your eyes and find the candle image imprinted on your eyelids. Stay with it.

5. As the image fades, open your eyes and see the candle again.

6. Continue for 15 to 20 minutes.

VISUALIZATION. Wherever you are, your mind can help you to substitute the pleasant for the unpleasant, to escape your present tension for a calmer place for a little while, leaving you feeling more relaxed and better able to cope when you return to reality.

1. Sit in a comfortable chair or lie down on your bed.

2. Close your eyes. Imagine that you are leaving the area where you are, leaving all the present hassles and pressures behind and arriving at another place. Where you choose to arrive depends on where you feel most relaxed—perhaps a deserted beach, a mountaintop, a garden, or beside a rippling stream or waterfall.

3. Take in every detail of your new surroundings, the colors, smells, and sounds. Remember just how you feel when you are in a place like this. Remember the feeling of the warm sun on your body, the caress of a soft breeze, the songs of the birds, the rush of the ocean, or running water. Enjoy the sensations of being there, of relaxing there.

4. After 3 to 5 minutes, take a long last look around you at your imaginary surroundings and then slowly open your eyes. You have created your own private escape, a place you can come back to whenever you need to relax.

YOGA. Yoga is slow and gentle exercise that stresses tension-reducing stretching and the kind of deep breathing that you learned about in the first exercise above. It should be done in a darkened room to a background of soft relaxing music and should end with total body relaxation. If yoga is practiced regularly, it will work like any good stretching exercise to help firm muscles and increase flexibility. The special advantage of this kind of exercise is its soothing, calming effect.

Here is a simple yoga routine you can practice at home. Remember to use slow and deliberate movements. Let the breathing take you into the stretch and emphasize holding the stretch, never bouncing. Each exercise should be held once for 10 seconds and then repeated two more times for a longer stretch each time, first for 15 and then for 20 seconds.

1. Stand with your knees slightly bent and your arms at your sides. Inhale, reach high for the ceiling, and hold. Exhale as your bring your arms down.

2. Standing with your arms at your sides, neck and chin down, bend your head first to the right shoulder and hold and then to the left.

3. Hold your arms out straight in front of your body. Flex your palms up, with your fingertips toward the ceiling, and then turn your palms down. Shift your arms straight out to the sides and repeat the palm movements, first up and then down.

4. Place your hands on your shoulders. Make forward circles with your elbows, then reverse. Move very slowly.

5. With your feet 6 inches apart, bring your left hand over your head, exhale and stretch over as far as you can toward the right. Return to the center and repeat the movement to the left, with your right hand over your head.

6. Step out with your right foot, inhale, move your left hand as far down as you can along your right leg toward the floor, bringing your right arm behind you into the air and looking up to your right hand. Repeat on the left, using the bottom hand to keep your balance.

7. Sit down on the floor with your back straight and the bottoms of your feet together; put your hands on your feet. Do a gentle up-and-down butterfly movement with your knees.

8. Still sitting on the floor with your back straight, spread your legs out, and breathe in deeply. Place your right hand behind your buttocks on the floor, exhale, and reach your left hand toward your right foot, dropping your head toward your right knee. Return to the first position and repeat the movements to the left.

9. Sit up again, bringing your legs together. Inhale and reach overhead. As you breathe out, reach toward your feet, bringing your head down toward the floor.

10. Sit up straight and cross your legs in the Indian position. Place your left hand on your right knee and your right hand on the floor behind your buttocks. Inhale, then, as you exhale, look over your right shoulder. Release and repeat with your right hand on your left knee, looking over your left shoulder.

11. Lie on your back, arms straight out to the sides. Bring your knees to your chest; then shift them over to the floor on the left, turning your head to the right. Reverse.

12. Still lying on your back, keep your left leg out straight and clasp your arms around your right knee. Release and reverse legs. Then bring both knees up and wrap your arms around your knees; grasp your elbows and hold for 10 seconds.

13. Lie on your back on the floor with both knees bent and your feet flat on the floor. Lift your left leg toward the ceiling, clasp your hands behind your left calf, and slowly stretch your right leg straight out on the floor. Return to the original position and alternate legs.

14. Conclude your yoga workout by lying on your back with your arms and legs relaxed. Close your eyes. Mentally move slowly up your body from your toes to your head—toes, feet, calves, knees, thighs, buttocks, stomach, chest, arms, shoulders, and head. As you reach each part, let it go limp and silently tell it to relax. When you reach the top of your body (your head), remain in this totally relaxed position for 5 minutes. Breathe deeply in and out, focusing your mind on the number one. If thoughts intrude, let them go and continue to concentrate only on the number one.

15. Very slowly open your eyes and tell your body to wake up, mentally working your way slowly up your body again. Roll over to the right into a fetal position and slowly resume a sitting position. Sit in a yoga Indian position with your legs crossed and clasp your hands behind your back. Inhale, then exhale, lowering your head toward the floor, and raise your arms behind you toward the ceiling. Return to the original position, reverse your legs, clasp your hands behind your back again, inhale, and as you exhale, drop your head again. Slowly stand—and go on your way, feeling refreshed and relaxed.

These are but a few of many yoga positions and routines. If you like the relaxed feeling and flexibility these exercises bring, find a book on yoga or join a class.

HELP FOR THE INSOMNIAC

Without a good night's sleep, it's difficult to meet life's demands. If you have problems sleeping, you are in good company, for a recent Gallup poll showed that 52 percent of the population suffers to some extent from insomnia. Regular exercise will help you sleep better. Here are a few other suggestions to help you get more rest.

WAYS TO PREPARE MIND AND BODY FOR RESTFUL SLEEP

- Retire at about the same time each night.
- Make sure the bedroom is quiet and dark.
- Keep the room cool and the air moist. A humidifier in winter can help.
- Prepare for bed in a leisurely manner—a warm bath and soft music are good presleep activities.
- A light snack before bed may help you sleep better, particularly a glass of lukewarm milk. But avoid caffeine in the evening.
- Don't bring work into the bedroom.
- Studies show that people who usually assume the same sleep position fall asleep more easily.
- Monotonous noise, such as rain on the roof, induces sleep. You can also buy "white noise machines," devices that give off soothing sounds.
- When you get into bed, concentrate on how tired you are. Try to blot out worries by visualizing a black dot or another neutral, pleasant mental image, or by counting backward from 100 very slowly.
- Breathe consciously in the sleep rhythm, using the deep-breathing techniques you learned above. Let the abdomen rise as you inhale and fall as you exhale.
- If you feel tension in your muscles, use progressive relaxation to ease it. Concentrate especially on relaxing your facial muscles.
- If you can't sleep, don't get uptight. Read a book, write a letter, or make a shopping list.

Mastering techniques for relaxing and sleeping is a step toward gaining more control over your life. Practicing them means you are beginning to take charge of your own well-being. A regular program of exercise and a healthful diet contribute to that well-being, as do strategies for improving your life. As your Palm-Aire Plan week ends, you will want to take concrete steps to continue the good start you have made this week, to ensure that your investment of time pays lifetime dividends.

10 WAYS TO REDUCE STRESS

1. Become more aware of the signals your body gives you about your inner reactions, both physical and emotional.

2. Gain more control over your life—start to create the kind of life you want, rather than just reacting to what seems to happen to you.

3. Learn techniques for relaxing the symptoms of stress.

4. Balance your work with plenty of time off for play.

5. Make time for regular exercise.

6. Eat a balanced diet and get enough rest.

7. Find a hobby that is creative rather than competitive. Gardening and painting are good examples.

8. Learn to work more constructively, finishing one task before starting another.

9. Express your feelings in a positive way—don't harbor antagonism or hostility.

10. Learn to like yourself better—look at your strengths as well as your weaknesses—and remember that everyone has weaknesses.

SUGGESTED READING

The Wellness Workbook by Regina Ryan and John Travis (Ten Speed Press, P.O. Box 7123, Berkeley, CA 94707).

The Relaxation & Stress Reduction Workbook by Martha Davis, Matthew McKay, and Elizabeth Robbins Eshelman (New Harbinger Publications, 2200 Adeline, Suite 305, Oakland, CA 94607).

SUGGESTED RECORDINGS FOR RELAXATION

Marcus Allen and Jon Bernoff, *Breathe* (Rising Sun Records, 158 E. Blithedale #4, Mill Valley, CA 94941).

Sri Chinmoy, *Music for Meditation* (Folkways 8935).

Environments Series, 10 discs with rain, surf, bird sounds, etc. (from Syntonic Research at 175 Fifth Ave., New York, NY 10010).

Wolff and Hennings, *Tibetan Bells* (Antilles 7006).

PIANO MUSIC

*Steve Bergman, *Music for an Inner Journey*.

*Steven Halpern, *Spectrum Suite, Starborn Suite, Zodiac Suite, Eastern Peace*, and others (Halpern Sounds, 620 Taylor Way #14, Belmont, CA 94002).

Keith Jarrett, *The Koln Concert* (ECM 1064/65).

HARP MUSIC

*Steven Halpern and Georgia Kelly, *Ancient Echoes*.

*Georgia Kelly, *Seapeace, Tarashanti, Birds of Paradise* (Heru, Box 954, Topanga, CA 90290).

FLUTE MUSIC

*Sach Dev, *Master of the Bamboo Flute*.

Paul Horn, *Inside* (in the Taj Mahal) (Epic 26466).

*Larkin, *To the Essence of a Candle: Wind Sung Sounds*.

GUITAR MUSIC

Robbie Basho, *Art of the Acoustic* (Windham Hill 1010).

Linda Cohen, *Angel Allen* (Tomato 7010).

*Alex DeGrassi, *Slow Circle* (Windham Hill 1009).

*William Eaton, *Music by William Eaton*.

*The complete list is available for $2 from Lloyd Barde, 4008 Idaho, Evan, CO, 80620.

A New Plan

Your Palm-Aire 7-Day Plan is over—and what have you accomplished? If you have been faithful, you've done far more than take off a few pounds.

You've begun to trim inches and make flabby muscles firmer. You've learned to replace sloppy skin and nail care habits with healthy ones and to make the most of your appearance. You've discovered smarter, more satisfying, yet delicious, menus and eating habits that can keep you trim for life. Along the way, you have also learned more about how your body works and how to help it, about how to strengthen your back and make your heart's work easier.

During this week, you've worked off a lot of tension with exercise. After the initial soreness and fatigue, you should have been rewarded also with the magical discovery that working hard actually generates new energy.

You've practiced other techniques that help you control the symptoms of tension and stress when they occur, and you've begun looking at your life to find ways of reducing the stresses and increasing the satisfactions.

Not bad for a week's investment of time. Right now you

173

should be sharing a lot of the good feeling that Spa-goers experience when their week is completed.

But, of course, it's after the week is over that the real test begins. This week should have proven to you that it *is* possible to change your life. You've seen that you can find the time for exercise if you want to badly enough, and that there are ways to lose weight yet eat satisfying meals. You've seen that small steps can bring big changes in your looks and outlook, and you've thought about constructive ways to change your life for the better.

While the glow of the Palm-Aire 7-Day Plan remains, make a new chart with targets for continuing your good start in the weeks ahead. In some ways, it will be much easier than during this past week, because you won't need as much time. You don't need three exercise sessions or a beauty treatment every day. A brisk half-hour's walk every other day is really all you need to reach your aerobic goals, and a home session or an exercise class three times a week will continue to firm your body as you lose weight.

What you will need most of all is structure, a schedule with definite segments of your time blocked out to do what is necessary to continue to lose weight, stay fit, and look your best. You need to set time aside for yourself as religiously as you set aside time for work or family.

Exercise is easier to stay with when you have company, so now is the time to join a health club, an exercise class, or the "Y" to help reinforce your good intentions. A club that offers many types of exercises makes it easy to vary your routine and keep it interesting. If you've also been meaning to learn a new sport, such as tennis or golf, sign up for lessons right now while your momentum is still in full gear. The exercise may not be aerobic, but it will still burn calories and help you control your weight while you have fun. A more active life-style is a more satisfying one, and the more ways you find to relax, the more you will enjoy life.

While your good intentions are strong, take advantage of this opportunity to look into other ways to make your life more rewarding, whether that means relaxing with yoga, finding confidence from assertiveness training, seeking reassurance in a support group, or undertaking study for a more satisfying career.

It's easier to take small steps toward change than giant ones, so when you write down your good intentions, do it according to priorities. The first priority is to continue your fitness program. It will make you look and feel better and give you the incentive to do more. In each life category, begin with your first goal and move on to the second only when number one has been accomplished.

Particularly where weight loss is concerned, for the best chance at success, keep your targets short term. Remember that stringent diets simply don't work in the long run, so make it easier on yourself by working toward small losses that will quickly add up—and last. For example, aim for 5 pounds off in the next 4 weeks, rather than setting your sights on a much harder-to-attain 20-pound weight loss. When you reach your 5-pound goal, reward yourself—not with food, but with tickets to a play or a new outfit to show off your slimmer shape. Then, reinforced by your success, set your new goal for the next 4 weeks.

Good things don't happen overnight, and your final fitness goals will not be reached quickly either. There is no instant gratification when it comes to fitness. It takes 3 months to see any really substantial results, so don't be discouraged. And don't give up if you have occasional lapses. The Spa philosophy is a positive one that you can share: Do your best, praise yourself when you do well, and try, try again when you don't. If you keep at it, you *will* succeed. Your habits will gradually change and you will begin to see these changes reflected in your own well-being.

The Palm-Aire 7-Day Plan is a quick start. It can prove to be a week that changes your life if you let these 7 days become the beginning of a more fulfilling future. Here are charts to keep track of your fitness progress and a personal goal chart. Use them as road maps to guide you to a happier, healthier way of life.

FITNESS RECORDS

	Miles walked	Aerobic exercise (minutes)	Calisthenics or other exercise (minutes)
Monday			
Tuesday			
Wednesday			
Thursday			
Friday			
Saturday			
Sunday			

	Week 1	Week 2	Week 3	Week 4	Week 5	Week 6
Aerobic time spent						
Exercise time						
Resting pulse rate						
Pulse rate during aerobic exercise						
Weight						
Measurements:						
Neck						
Upper arm						
Forearm						
Chest						
Bust						
Diaphragm						
Waist						
Abdomen						
Hip						
Thigh						
Calf						
Knee						

MY PERSONAL GOALS (SAMPLE CHART)

Exercise goals

1. Aerobic exercise at least 3 times a week.

2. Enroll in a calisthenics class.

3. Learn to play tennis.

In order to accomplish these goals, I must do the following:

1. Set aside the following times for the following aerobics:
Monday, Noon: 1 hour walk
Tuesday
Wednesday, 6 P.M.: *Aerobic dance class*
Thursday
Friday: Either lunchtime walk or additional 6 P.M. *dance class*
Saturday
Sunday, 2 P.M.: *Bike ride*

2. Get prices and time schedules and visit a few potential exercise classes to choose the place I am most likely to enjoy. Sign up.

3. Get prices of tennis lessons and look at facilities. Sign up for a series of lessons.

Diet goals

1. I will lose _____ pounds in the next _____ weeks.

In order to accomplish these goals, I must do the following:

1. Change my snacking habits.

2. Cut down portions.

3. Modify recipes to use less fat and sugar.

4. Drink more water to help my body's processes work smoothly.

Grooming goals

1. I will give myself a facial masque treatment at home once a week.

2. I will give myself a weekly manicure.

3. I will have a professional facial once a month.

4. I will find a better hairdresser.

In order to accomplish these goals, I must do the following:

1. Set aside every Monday evening for a facial and manicure.

2. Phone to check prices, book a facial at a different place for each of the next 3 months, then sign up for a series at the place I like best.

3. Ask friends for recommendations of hairdressers and try a new one the next time I need a haircut, being very specific about what I want.

Life-style goals

1. More free time for fun.

2. More friends.

3. A more positive outlook.

4. A more rewarding job.

In order to accomplish these goals, I must do the following:

1. Look at my daily and weekly routines to see where I am spending time least productively, and cut out those activities.

2. Stop staying at the office past 5:15.

3. Take up tennis and join a club.

4. Practice stress-reduction routines.

5. Join a group for single parents.

6. Put my résumé in order and begin a serious job search.

MY PERSONAL GOALS

Exercise goals

1. ....

2. ....

3. ....

4. ....

In order to accomplish these goals, I must do the following:

1. ....

2. ....

3. ....

4. ....

Diet goals

1. ....

2. ....

In order to accomplish these goals, I must do the following:

1. ....

2. ....

3. ....

4. ....

Grooming goals

1. ....

2. ....

3. ....

4. ....

In order to accomplish these goals, I must do the following:

1. ....

2. ....

3. ....

4. ....

Life-style goals

1. ....

2. ....

3. ....

4. ....

In order to accomplish these goals, I must do the following:

1. ....

2. ....

3. ....

4. ....

Other goals

1. ....
2. ....
3. ....
4. ....

In order to accomplish these goals, I must do the following:

1. ....
2. ....
3. ....
4. ....

The Palm-Aire Recipe Book

On the Palm-Aire Plan, the emphasis is not on dieting but on eating—and eating well. At the Spa, the secret to losing weight is not doing without, but doing differently—choosing the kinds of foods that let you enjoy eating while you are controlling your calorie intake.

The following week of recipes from Palm-Aire will give you a taste of the Spa menu, a variety of dishes that are low in calories but high in nutrition, variety, and taste appeal.

This is not a fad diet to follow for a week and forget, but an introduction to a way of healthy eating that can be part of your life forever. Each meal is planned to give the variety of elements a balanced diet requires, including carbohydrates, protein, and fiber, and to be low in fats as well. Each meal includes several courses of sensible, small portions designed to send you away from the table feeling satisfied.

At Palm-Aire a variety of food is stressed while you are counting calories, because without it, it is only natural to crave the foods you are denied. So these menus call for many different kinds of foods each day, and a sweet ending to stave off that familiar yearning when desserts are denied.

If you follow this regimen as it is served at the Spa, you will go without caffeine and salt for this week—and you may be surprised to discover how little you miss them. Each meal offers a choice of decaffeinated coffee or rose hips tea, served hot or cold. Use Mrs. Dash, the seasoning Spa guests find on the table with the pepper shaker instead of salt, and experiment with flavorings, such as garlic and onion powder, and herbs, such as marjoram, basil, and tarragon, to add flavor to your food without adding salt.

The calorie count each day varies from 800 to 1,000 calories, because the Palm-Aire philosophy is that variety is more important than counting exact calories. You'll notice that the calories are distributed to provide a substantial breakfast and lunch each day. Skipping or skimping on a meal to save calories is a common mistake. By providing calories when the body needs them for energy to keep going all day, you will not gain weight—and you will be less likely to overeat at dinner.

Spa guests who follow this menu usually lose from 5 to 7 pounds in a week. After the first week, the goal should be only 1 to 2 pounds a week, because only pounds shed in a slow sustained manner will stay off permanently. To continue to lose, you need only follow the basic Palm-Aire formula—high carbohydrate, medium protein, and low fat. If you do, you will find you can enjoy your meals and still lose weight.

Here are basic menus for 7 days. Every attempt has been made to adapt these recipes to ingredients easily accessible at home, which often means taking advantage of prepared low-calorie products. If you try several bottled low-calorie salad dressings, you may find one you particularly enjoy. You will find recipes for homemade dressings at the end of the section.

The actual Spa menu includes several substitute choices available every day for breakfast and lunch, and those choices also have been included at the end of the section, along with a few quick-to-make substitute dinners to please varying tastes.

Many Spa dessert recipes use low-calorie whipped toppings, such as Dream Whip. Because these cannot easily be made in small servings, you may choose to alter the menus and repeat some desserts rather than let them go to waste. The calorie counts for all desserts are identical.

You can also make use of other low-calorie prepared desserts, such as frozen yogurt, ice milk, and frozen fruit bars to vary your menus. A serving of ¼ cup will satisfy your sweet tooth without spoiling your weight loss. Again, the variety and the satisfaction are more important than an extra 20 or 30 calories a day.

Snacks are allowed on the Palm-Aire Plan—as long as they are fresh fruit and vegetables. Follow what is done at the Spa and have a ready supply of these on hand to fight the temptation to reach for more fattening things when the snack urge strikes.

Remember one other important Spa secret: When you prepare meals, garnish each dish to make it look as attractive as you can. Even the simplest salad can seem special and appetizing when prepared with care. If you take the trouble to make the meal look appealing and make the time to sit down and enjoy each course, you will feel less of a craving for more food afterward. Try it and see for yourself.

DAY I: MENUS

Breakfast	Calories
4 ounces fruit juice	40
Jarlsberg Egg White Omelet	75
1 slice whole wheat toast	70
Decaffeinated coffee or rose hips tea	0
	185

Lunch	Calories
Beef Consommé Celestine	40
Broccoli, Cauliflower, and Carrot Salad	20
Chicken Chow Mein with Chinese noodles	175
Chocolate–Peppermint Mousse	40
Decaffeinated coffee or rose hips tea	0
	275

Dinner	Calories
Artichoke Hearts Vinaigrette	40
Romaine Salad	20
Tenderloin Kabob over rice	200
½ cup steamed carrots	20
Light Cheesecake	40
Decaffeinated coffee or rose hips tea	0
	320

DAY I: RECIPES

Jarlsberg Egg White Omelet

MAKES 1 SERVING (75 CALORIES)

2 egg whites
½ ounce Jarlsberg cheese, shredded
Vegetable cooking spray (Pam)

Beat the egg whites as you would for an omelet, then fold in the cheese. Pour into a preheated frying pan sprayed with cooking spray and cook over medium heat until the bottom of the omelet is firm. Fold the omelet in half, and cook for a few moments longer to allow time for the cheese to melt completely. Remove from the heat and serve.

Beef Consommé Celestine

MAKES 1 SERVING (40 CALORIES)

¾ *cup beef stock skimmed of fat (low-sodium packaged bouillon cubes or broth may be used)*
4 to 5 eggless noodles (pasta)
Chopped fresh parsley leaves
Mrs. Dash seasoning mix

Put the beef stock and noodles in a saucepan. Bring to a boil, cover, and simmer over very low heat for 15 to 25 minutes, until liquid is reduced to ½ cup. Add the chopped parsley and Mrs. Dash to taste.

Broccoli, Cauliflower, and Carrot Salad

MAKES 1 SERVING (20 CALORIES)

1 small carrot, sliced
1 broccoli floret
1 cauliflower floret
1 lettuce leaf
Thin slice of pimiento,
1 tablespoon low-calorie salad dressing

Arrange the carrot slices and cauliflower and broccoli florets attractively on the lettuce leaf. Garnish with the pimiento slice. Drizzle with the salad dressing before serving.

Chicken Chow Mein

MAKES 1 SERVING (175 CALORIES)

Vegetable cooking spray (Pam)
3 ounces boneless and skinless chicken breast
¾ cup mixed Chinese vegetables (may include baby corn, water chestnuts, bamboo shoots, straw mushrooms, leeks, bean sprouts, snow peas, Chinese cabbage, and black mushrooms)
½ cup low-sodium chicken stock
2 teaspoons arrowroot
1 teaspoon teriyaki sauce
Garlic powder, ground ginger, Mrs. Dash seasoning mix, and white pepper to taste
¼ cup Chinese noodles

Spray a frying pan with the cooking spray. Heat the pan and fry the chicken until it is cooked. Add the vegetables and chicken stock and sauté until the vegetables are just crisp. Add the arrowroot slowly to thicken sauce; then bring to a simmer and add the teriyaki sauce and seasonings to taste. Serve with the noodles.

Chocolate-Peppermint Mousse	MAKES 4 SERVINGS (40 CALORIES EACH)

Chocolate-Peppermint Mousse

MAKES 4 SERVINGS (40 CALORIES EACH)

½ package (¾ ounce) Dream Whip
1 tablespoon diet chocolate pudding powder
¼ teaspoon peppermint extract
1 egg white, beaten until stiff
4 fresh mint leaves

Prepare the Dream Whip following the package directions. Add the pudding powder and peppermint extract and beat the mixture with an electric mixer for 1 minute. Fold in the beaten egg whites. Chill well before serving. Garnish with fresh mint leaves.

Artichoke Hearts Vinaigrette

MAKES 1 SERVING (40 CALORIES)

2 canned artichoke hearts, drained and halved
low-calorie Italian salad dressing
Chopped parsley
Lemon wedge

Marinate the artichoke hearts in the diet dressing for 2 hours. Remove from the dressing and place on a lettuce leaf. Garnish with the chopped parsley and a lemon wedge.

Romaine Salad

MAKES 1 SERVING (20 CALORIES)

2 cherry tomatoes
1 cup chopped romaine Lettuce
1 tablespoon low-calorie salad dressing

Put the tomatoes on the lettuce in a salad bowl. Drizzle with the salad dressing before serving.

Tenderloin Kabobs

MAKES 4 SERVINGS (200 CALORIES EACH)

12 ounces beef tenderloin, cut into 1-ounce cubes
1 medium-size onion, cut into eighths
1 sweet green pepper, cut into eighths
8 large fresh mushroom caps
8 small clusters fresh broccoli
1 cup hot cooked rice

On each of 4 skewers, arrange 3 cubes of tenderloin and 2 wedges of each vegetable. Broil for 7 to 12 minutes, turning occasionally. Serve hot over ¼ cup of the rice.

**Light
Cheesecake**

MAKES 6 SERVINGS (40 CALORIES EACH)

1½ *tablespoons unflavored gelatin*
¼ *cup canned unsweetened pineapple juice, heated*
¼ *cup unsweetened shredded coconut*
1 *cup prepared Dream Whip*
¼ *cup canned, unsweetened pineapple chunks*
1 *packet Sweet 'n Low*
1½ *cups lowfat cottage cheese, puréed*

Dissolve the gelatin in the hot pineapple juice. Add the coconut and chill until firm, but not completely set. Prepare the Dream Whip following the package directions; then fold in the pineapple and Sweet 'n Low and set aside. Combine the gelatin mixture with the puréed cottage cheese. Beat at medium speed with an electric mixer for 2 to 3 minutes. Fold in the Dream Whip mixture at low speed until blended. Pour into an 8-inch square pan. Chill for at least 2 hours before serving.

DAY II: MENUS

Breakfast	Calories
½ grapefruit	40
Strawberry Crêpes with Mock Sour Cream	200
Decaffeinated coffee or rose hips tea	0
	240

Lunch	Calories
3 ounces cranberry juice	40
Garden Salad	20
Fettuccine Marco	175
Applesauce Pudding	40
Decaffeinated coffee or rose hips tea	0
	275

Dinner	Calories
Zucchini Consommé	40
Lettuce wedge with lemon	20
Chicken Cacciatore served with rice	175
½ cup steamed broccoli	20
Pineapple–Coconut Bavarian	40
Decaffeinated coffee or rose hips tea	0
	295

DAY II: RECIPES

Crêpes

MAKES 10 CRÊPES (APPROXIMATELY 70 CALORIES EACH)

½ cup whole wheat flour
¼ teaspoon salt
5 egg whites
1 cup skim or lowfat buttermilk
½ cup plus 1 tablespoon safflower oil

Combine the dry ingredients in a bowl. Beat the egg whites until fluffy. Stir the milk and oil into the egg whites. Add the liquids to the flour mixture and stir until smooth. The batter will be thin. Drop on a preheated nonstick griddle, using about 1½ ounces (3 tablespoons) for each crêpe. Brown lightly on both sides. The crêpes will roll more easily if they are not overcooked. Any crêpes not served immediately can be frozen. Stack with wax paper between each crêpe to prevent sticking, wrap securely, and freeze until needed.

Strawberry Crêpes

MAKES 1 SERVING (200 CALORIES)

½ cup cut up strawberries
2 crêpes
Mock Sour Cream (made from 2 ounces lowfat yogurt flavored with lemon juice to taste)

Put ¼ cup of the strawberries on each crêpe, roll the crêpe up, and cover with the mock sour cream.

Garden Salad

MAKES 1 SERVING (20 CALORIES)

1 cup mixed iceberg and romaine lettuce
¼ cup shredded carrot and summer squash, mixed
1 tomato wedge
1 tablespoon low-calorie salad dressing

Put the lettuce in a small bowl and top with the shredded vegetables and tomato wedge. Drizzle with the salad dressing before serving.

Fettuccine Marco

MAKES 4 SERVINGS (175 CALORIES EACH)
1 cup (¼ pound) uncooked fettuccine
4 ounces part-skim ricotta cheese
4 egg whites
8 ounces plain lowfat yogurt
4 tablespoons grated Parmesan cheese
4 parsley sprigs

Preheat the oven to 325 degrees. Cook the fettuccine in a large pot of boiling water until it is *al dente* (soft but still firm). Drain the cooked fettuccine and run it under cold water until it is chilled; drain well. Using an electric mixer, whip the ricotta cheese, egg whites, and yogurt together until smooth. Combine this mixture with the drained fettuccine in a small casserole dish and sprinkle the Parmesan cheese on top. Bake for 15 minutes. Cut into 4 equal portions, garnish with a parsley sprig, and serve hot.

Applesauce Pudding

MAKES 4 SERVINGS (40 CALORIES EACH)
1 egg white, beaten until stiff
½ cup prepared Dream Whip
¼ medium-size apple, cored
¼ teaspoon ground cinnamon
¼ teaspoon ground nutmeg

Put the apple, nutmeg, and cinnamon in a blender and purée until smooth. Fold the purée into the prepared Dream Whip; then fold in the egg whites. Chill until ready to serve.

Zucchini Consommé

MAKES 1 SERVING (40 CALORIES)
¾ cup low-sodium chicken stock
⅓ cup shredded zucchini
Mrs. Dash seasoning mix

Bring the stock to a boil, cover, and simmer over very low heat for 15 to 25 minutes, until liquid is reduced to ½ cup. Add the zucchini and reheat. Season with Mrs. Dash to taste.

Chicken Cacciatore

MAKES 4 SERVINGS (175 CALORIES EACH)
4 4-ounce chicken breasts, skinned
½ cup chopped scallion tops
½ cup chopped sweet green pepper
1 large tomato, diced

½ *cup water or low-sodium chicken stock*
½ *teaspoon dried oregano*
½ *teaspoon black pepper*
2 *garlic cloves, crushed and peeled*
1 *bay leaf*
1 *cup unsalted tomato juice*
2 *cups hot cooked rice*

Braise the chicken breasts and vegetables over low heat in a nonstick skillet with the water or chicken stock until the chicken is just tender. Mix the seasonings and tomato juice together in a bowl. Pour the mixture over chicken breast and vegetables, cover, and simmer for 20 to 25 minutes. Place each serving over ½ cup rice.

Pineapple-Coconut Bavarian

MAKES 6 SERVINGS (40 CALORIES EACH)
2 *egg whites*
½ *teaspoon cream of tartar*
1 *envelope Dream Whip*
6 *teaspoons puréed unsweetened pineapple, canned or fresh*
1 *teaspoon unsweetened shredded coconut*
1 *tablespoon Siba Pineapple-Coconut Delight (piña colada mix)*

Beat the egg whites and cream of tartar with an electric mixer until stiff peaks form. Prepare Dream Whip following the package directions and add the Pineapple–Coconut Delight. Fold the egg whites into the Dream Whip mixture. Transfer to a serving dish and chill for 1 hour before serving. Spoon 1 teaspoon of pineapple purée over each portion and garnish with some shredded coconut.

DAY III: MENUS

Breakfast	Calories
½ banana	50
Buckwheat Pancakes with Blueberries	200
Decaffeinated coffee or rose hips tea	0
	250

Lunch	Calories
Consommé au Sherry	40
Coleslaw	20
Tuna Salad Sandwich in Pita Bread	175
Apple Snow	40
Decaffeinated coffee or rose hips tea	0
	275

Dinner	Calories
Stuffed Mushrooms	20
Beet and Onion Salad	20
Veal Florentine served with half a baked potato	200
1/2 cup steamed cauliflower	20
Peach Fluff	40
Decaffeinated coffee or rose hips tea	0
	300

DAY III: RECIPES

Buckwheat Pancakes with Blueberries

MAKES 10 PANCAKES, 5 SERVINGS (200 CALORIES EACH)

2 egg whites, slightly beaten
1 cup skim milk
1 1/2 cups whole wheat flour
1 teaspoon baking powder
2 1/2 cups cooked blueberries

Combine the milk and egg whites in a bowl. Sift the flour and baking powder together and stir into milk mixture until moistened. Drop the batter onto a heated nonstick griddle. Cook until bubbles appear; then turn and cook on the other side. Serve warm with 1/4 cup cooked blueberries on each pancake.

Consommé au Sherry

MAKES 6 SERVINGS (40 CALORIES EACH)

4 cups low-sodium chicken broth
1/2 cup cooking sherry
1 garlic clove, crushed and peeled
2 tablespoons dried parsley flakes or chopped fresh parsley leaves

Combine all the ingredients in a 2-quart saucepan. Bring to a boil and simmer for 15 to 20 minutes.

Coleslaw	MAKES 4 SERVINGS (20 CALORIES EACH) 1½ *cups shredded white cabbage* ½ *cup shredded carrot* 1 *tablespoon celery seed* *Mustard Sauce (recipe below) to taste* Mix all the ingredients together in a bowl. For better taste, cover and refrigerate several hours.
Mustard Sauce	MAKES 1 CUP (20 CALORIES PER TBSP.) ¾ *cup low-calorie salad dressing* ¼ *cup Dijon mustard* Combine the ingredients in a bowl and mix well.
Tuna Salad Sandwich in Pita Bread	MAKES 1 SERVING (175 CALORIES) 3 *ounces water-packed canned white tuna* 1 *tablespoon low-calorie salad dressing* ½ *cup chopped celery, onion, and carrot, mixed* ½ *pita bread* 1 *lettuce leaf* 1 *tomato slice* Mix the tuna, salad dressing, and vegetables together in a bowl. Transfer to the pita bread pocket. Serve with a lettuce leaf and a slice of tomato.
Apple Snow	MAKES 4 SERVINGS (40 CALORIES EACH) 1 *egg white* ¼ *teaspoon cream of tartar* ½ *cup Dream Whip* 1½ *tablespoons unsweetened apple juice* ¼ *cup puréed unpeeled Red Delicious apple* ¼ *teaspoon ground cinnamon* Beat the egg white and cream of tartar with an electric mixer at high speed until stiff peaks form. Set aside. Prepare the Dream Whip following the package directions, substituting the apple juice and puréed apple for ¼ cup of the liquid called for. Add cinnamon. Fold the beaten egg white into the Dream Whip mixture. Spoon into serving glasses and chill for at least 1 hour before serving.

Stuffed Mushrooms

MAKES 6 SERVINGS (40 CALORIES EACH)

1/4 *medium-size onion*
1/8 *cup Miller's bran (unprocessed bran)*
1/2 *celery stalk*
1/4 *cup skim milk*
2 *ounces crab meat, fresh, frozen, or canned*
2 *teaspoons Vegit Vegetable Seasoning*
12 *large fresh mushroom caps*

Preheat the oven to 350 degrees. Put all the ingredients, except the mushrooms, into a food processor or blender and blend well. Stuff the mushrooms with the mixture and put them in a small baking pan. Bake for 10 to 15 minutes, or until the tops are browned. Serve immediately.

Beet and Onion Salad

MAKES 1 SERVING (20 CALORIES)

1/4 *cup sliced cooked beets*
1 *slice onion*
2 *tablespoons red wine vinegar*
1 *lettuce leaf*

Combine all the ingredients in a bowl and let stand for 1 hour. Serve on the lettuce leaf.

Veal Florentine

MAKES 4 SERVINGS (200 *calories each*)

4 2 1/2-*ounce veal cutlets*
1 *cup low-sodium chicken broth*
1 *tablespoon arrowroot*
2 *ounces cooked spinach*
2 *hot baked potatoes, cut in half lengthwise*
1 *tablespoon chopped fresh parsley leaves*
Mrs. Dash seasoning mix

Pound the veal with a flat mallet to a 1/2-inch thickness. Put the veal, 1/2 cup of the chicken broth, and the seasonings in a frying pan. Cover and cook over low heat until the veal is barely tender. Mix the arrowroot with the remaining 1/2 cup of broth and stir into the veal mixture. Add the spinach and simmer for 20 to 30 minutes, or until the veal can be cut with a fork. Adjust the seasonings and serve hot with half of a baked potato.

Peach Fluff   MAKES 4 SERVINGS (40 CALORIES EACH)
½ tablespoon low-calorie peach-flavored gelatin powder
¼ cup puréed fresh peach
½ cup boiling water
1 cup prepared Dream Whip

Dissolve the gelatin and puréed peach in the boiling water. Chill until set. When the gelatin mixture is firm, beat it with an electric mixer until it has doubled in volume. Fold in the Dream Whip. Spoon into serving glasses and chill for at least 1 hour.

DAY IV: MENUS

Breakfast	Calories
½ cup fresh strawberries	50
1 Bran Muffin	75
¼ cup lowfat cottage cheese	40
Decaffeinated coffee or rose hips tea	0
	165

Lunch	Calories
Gazpacho	40
Bibb Lettuce Salad	20
Herbed Baked Fish Fillets served with rice	175
Fruit Cup	75
	310

Dinner	Calories
Hearts of Palm	40
Garden Salad	20
Fettuccine with Seafood Marinara	175
½ cup steamed green beans	20
Baked Almond Apple	40
	295

DAY IV: RECIPES

Bran Muffins

MAKES 12 MUFFINS (75 CALORIES EACH)
½ cup whole wheat flour
½ cup unprocessed bran flakes
2 tablespoons baking powder
¼ cup finely diced apple
1 teaspoon ground cinnamon
½ teaspoon ground nutmeg
½ cup boiling water
1 egg, beaten
1 tablespoon safflower oil
¼ cup blackstrap molasses
¼ cup honey
¾ cup skim buttermilk
Vegetable cooking spray (Pam)

Combine the flour, bran flakes, and baking powder in a large bowl. In a separate bowl, mix the apple, cinnamon, nutmeg, and boiling water together; refrigerate until cool. Preheat the oven to 325 degrees. Then combine the beaten egg, oil, molasses, honey, buttermilk, and apple mixture with the dry ingredients and gently fold them together. Portion into a lightly sprayed muffin tin. Bake for 35 minutes. The muffins may be frozen.

Gazpacho

MAKES 4 SERVINGS (40 CALORIES EACH)
3 6-ounce cans low-sodium V-8 juice
⅓ cup chopped cucumber
⅓ cup chopped sweet green pepper
⅓ cup chopped onion

Combine all the ingredients in blender and purée until smooth. Transfer to a bowl, cover, and chill before serving.

Bibb Lettuce Salad

MAKES 1 SERVING (20 CALORIES)
½ cup shredded Bibb lettuce
Sliced onion
Shredded carrot
2 cherry tomatoes
1 tablespoon low-calorie salad dressing

Combine all the ingredients in a bowl. Drizzle with the salad dressing before serving.

194

Herbed Baked Fish Fillets	MAKES 4 SERVINGS (175 CALORIES EACH)

Herbed Baked Fish Fillets

MAKES 4 SERVINGS (175 CALORIES EACH)

½ cup whole wheat flour
½ teaspooon garlic powder
½ teaspoon dried oregano
1 teaspoon grated fresh ginger
1 to 1½ pounds fish fillets
1 egg white, lightly beaten
½ cup plain lowfat yogurt
2 cups hot cooked rice

Preheat the oven to 400 degrees. Combine the flour, garlic powder, oregano, and ginger. Dip the fish in egg white and then coat it with the flour mixture. Place fish in single layer in a baking pan. Spoon the yogurt over the fillets and bake for 15 minutes. Serve each portion with ½ cup rice.

Fruit Cup

MAKES 1 SERVING (40 CALORIES)

Mix together ½ cup of seasonal fresh fruit, such as orange, grapefruit, pineapple, canteloupe, honeydew melon, or strawberries.

Hearts of Palm

MAKES 1 SERVING (40 CALORIES)

2 canned hearts of palm
1 teaspoon tarragon vinegar
2 lettuce leaves
Chopped fresh basil and parsley leaves

Thoroughly wash the can liquid from the hearts of palm. Cut the spears down the middle. Place 2 spears on each lettuce leaf. Season with vinegar, basil, and parsley.

Garden Salad

See recipe p. 187.

**Fettuccine
with Seafood
Marinara**

MAKES 4 SERVINGS (175 CALORIES EACH)

1/4 *cup low-sodium chicken broth*
1 *small onion, diced*
1 *garlic clove, crushed and peeled*
3/4 *cup low-sodium tomato sauce*
1 *teaspoon dry mustard*
4 *tablespoons fresh lemon juice*
1/2 *teaspoon chopped fresh oregano*
1 *pound seafood (use a combination of lobster, scallops, and crab meat)*
1 *cup (1/4 pound) uncooked fettuccine*

Combine all the ingredients, except the seafood mixture, in a saucepan; simmer, uncovered, for 20 minutes. Pour the sauce over the seafood and refrigerate for at least 1 hour. Broil for 8 to 12 minutes, turning occasionally and brushing frequently with the sauce. DO NOT OVERCOOK. Serve on 1/2 cup cooked fettuccine.

**Baked Almond
Apples**

MAKES 6 SERVINGS (40 CALORIES EACH)

3 *Red Delicious apples, cored and halved*
2 *tablespoons brown sugar*
2 *cups water*
1 *teaspoon ground cinnamon*
1/4 *teaspoon ground nutmeg*
1 *teaspoon almond extract*

Preheat the oven to 350 degrees. Place the apple halves cut side down in a baking pan. Mix the remaining ingredients together and pour over the apples. Bake for 40 minutes. Serve warm or chilled.

DAY V: MENUS

Breakfast	Calories
½ melon, any kind	50
French Toast with Apples	200
Decaffeinated coffee or rose hips tea	0
	250

Lunch	Calories
Leek Soup	40
Tomato and Onion Salad	20
Stuffed Zucchini with Fiber Dressing	175
Lemon Sponge	40
	275

Dinner	Calories
Seafood Cocktail	40
String Bean and Mushroom Salad	20
Marinated Flank Steak served with boiled potatoes	200
Steamed Mixed Vegetables	20
Strawberry Tart	40
	320

DAY V: RECIPES

French Toast with Apples

MAKES 1 SERVING (200 CALORIES)

2 egg whites
¼ cup lowfat milk
½ teaspoon vanilla extract
½ teaspoon ground cinnamon
2 slices bread
½ cup cooked unsweetened apples

Beat the egg whites until frothy; then beat in the milk powder, vanilla, and cinnamon. Dip the bread into the mixture to coat both sides. Place on a rack under a heated broiler and broil each side for about 3 minutes, or brown on a nonstick griddle. Serve hot with the apples spooned on top.

Leek Soup

6 cups low-sodium chicken broth
1 cup fresh leeks, cut into 1-inch slices and washed well
1 garlic clove, crushed
½ teaspoon black pepper
½ teaspoon arrowroot
1 teaspoons Vegit Vegetable Seasoning

Combine all the ingredients in a saucepan, bring to a boil, and simmer for 20 minutes. Serve hot.

Tomato and Onion Salad

MAKES 1 SERVING (20 CALORIES)
3 ¼-inch-thick tomato slices
Lettuce or other greens
2 ⅛-inch-thick onion slices
1 tablespoon low-calorie salad dressing

Put the tomato slices on a bed of lettuce and top with the onion slices. Chill well. Drizzle with the salad dressing before serving.

Stuffed Zucchini with Fiber Dressing

MAKES 2 SERVINGS (175 CALORIES EACH)
2 zucchini
Fiber dressing (recipe on facing page)
Vegetable cooking spray (Pam)

Preheat the oven to 350 degrees. Cut each zucchini in half lengthwise and scoop out the centers. Stuff each with ¼ cup of the Fiber Dressing and put them in a lightly sprayed baking pan. Bake for 20 minutes.

Fiber Dressing	MAKES 8 SERVINGS (APPROXIMATELY 25 CALORIES EACH)

½ *cup diced celery*
½ *cup diced onion*
½ *cup diced carrot*
1 *garlic clove, pressed*
½ *cup finely chopped fresh mushrooms*
1 *teaspoon chopped fresh parsley leaves*
½ *teaspoon herb seasoning*
½ *cup low-sodium chicken broth*
2 *egg whites*
4 *slices whole grain bread, diced*

Steam the vegetables and seasonings in the chicken broth for 8 to 10 minutes. Remove and combine with the egg whites and diced bread. Mix until all the ingredients are evenly blended. Refrigerate the leftovers for use on Day VI, in the stuffed chicken recipe.

Lemon Sponge	MAKES 2 SERVINGS (40 CALORIES EACH)

2 *egg whites*
½ *teaspoon cream of tartar*
½ *teaspoon lemon extract*
1 *cup prepared Dream Whip*

Beat the egg whites and cream of tartar with an electric mixer at high speed until stiff peaks form. Add the lemon extract to the Dream Whip and fold in the egg whites. Spoon into serving dishes and chill for at least 1 hour.

Seafood Cocktail	MAKES 1 SERVING (40 CALORIES)

1 *ounce poached seafood (use crab meat, shrimp, or lobster)*
Lettuce or other greens
2 *tablespoons Cocktail Sauce (recipe on next page)*
Lemon wedge

Put the seafood on a bed of greens and top with the sauce. Serve garnished with the lemon wedge.

Cocktail Sauce

MAKES 1 ½ CUPS (APPROXIMATELY 16 CALORIES PER OUNCE)

1 *cup low-sodium tomato juice*
¼ *cup bottled horseradish*
2 *tablespoons fresh lemon juice*
¼ *cup unsweetened pineapple juice*

Mix all the ingredients together, cover, and chill well before serving.

String Bean and Mushroom Salad

MAKES 1 SERVING (20 CALORIES)

½ *cup cut green beans and mushrooms, mixed*
Mustard Sauce (recipe below)
Lettuce or other greens

Put the beans and mushrooms on a bed of greens and top with 2 tablespoons of the mustard sauce.

Mustard Sauce

MAKES ¼ CUP (20 CALORIES PER TBSP.)

¼ *cup low-calorie prepared whipped salad dressing (D'Mayo or Weight Watchers)*
1 ½ *tablespoons cup Dijon mustard*

Combine the ingredients in a bowl and mix well. Chill before serving.

Marinated Flank Steak

MAKES 4 SERVINGS (200 CALORIES EACH)

10 *ounces flank steak*
½ *cup low-calorie French dressing*
Dash of black pepper
Vegetable cooking spray (Pam)
2 *cups hot boiled parsleyed potatoes*

Marinate the flank steak in the salad dressing and pepper in the refrigerator for 1 hour. Lightly spray a frying pan and cook the steak to taste. Serve with ½ cup boiled parsleyed potatoes.

Steamed Mixed Vegetables	MAKES 1 SERVING (20 CALORIES)

½ cup of any combination of the following vegetables:
  broccoli
  carrots
  cauliflower
  summer squash
  string beans
½ cup low-sodium chicken broth
Chopped fresh basil, fresh lemon juice, or Mrs. Dash seasoning mix

Steam the vegetables in the chicken broth until they are soft but still slightly crunchy. Season the stock with the basil, lemon juice, or Mrs. Dash to enhance the flavor.

Strawberry Dream

MAKES 4 SERVINGS (40 CALORIES EACH)

½ tablespoon low-calorie strawberry-flavored gelatin powder
¼ cup puréed strawberries
½ cup boiling water
1 cup prepared Dream Whip

Dissolve the gelatin and puréed strawberries in the boiling water. Chill until set. When gelatin mixture is firm, beat it with an electric mixer or egg beater until it has doubled in volume. Fold in the Dream Whip. Spoon into serving dishes and chill for at least 1 hour.

DAY VI: MENUS

Breakfast	**Calories**
Fruit Cup	40
Bagel Melt	200
Decaffeinated coffee or rose hips tea	0
	240

Lunch	**Calories**
Pineapple Suprême	40
Broccoli, Mushroom, and Carrot Curl Salad with Yogurt–Pineapple Dressing	20
Vegetable Lasagne	175
Cinnamon Mousse	40
Decaffeinated coffee or rose hips tea	0
	275

Dinner	Calories
Liver Pâté	40
Shredded Carrot Salad	20
Stuffed Chicken Suprême	200
½ cup steamed asparagus	20
Apricot Snow	40
Decaffeinated coffee or rose hips tea	0
	320

DAY VI: RECIPES

Fruit Cup

MAKES 1 SERVING (40 CALORIES)

Mix together ½ cup of seasonal fresh fruit, such as orange, grapefruit, pineapple, cantaloupe, honeydew melon, and strawberries.

Bagel Melt

MAKES 1 SERVING (200 CALORIES)
½ ounce Jarlsberg cheese, sliced
½ bagel, sliced in half
1 thin tomato slice

Lay the cheese slices on the bagel slices and broil for 1 minute, or until the cheese has melted. Garnish with the tomato slices.

Pineapple Suprême

MAKES 2 SERVINGS (40 CALORIES)
2 slices unsweetened canned pineapple
1 lettuce leaf
2 ounces lowfat cottage cheese

Put the pineapple on a lettuce leaf and top with the cottage cheese.

Broccoli, Mushroom, and Carrot Curl Salad

MAKES 1 SERVING (20 CALORIES)

1 *large fresh mushroom, sliced*
1 *carrot curl, 3 to 4 inches long*
1 *broccoli floret*
1 *lettuce leaf*
Pimiento slice
1 *tablespoon low-calorie salad dressing*

Arrange the vegetables on the lettuce and garnish with the pimiento. Drizzle with the salad dressing before serving.

Vegetable Lasagna

MAKES 4 SERVINGS (175 CALORIES EACH)

6 *uncooked lasagna noodles*
Vegetable cooking spray (Pam)
½ *cup diced onion*
½ *cup diced sweet green pepper*
½ *cup sliced fresh mushrooms*
12 *ounces low-sodium tomato sauce*
½ *cup steamed cauliflower*
½ *cup steamed zucchini*
½ *cup steamed broccoli*
½ *cup steamed summer squash*
4 *ounces part-skim ricotta cheese*
2 *ounces part-skim mozzarella cheese*

Cook the lasagna following the package directions until it is *al dente* (soft enough to eat but still firm in texture). Preheat the oven to 350 degrees. Spray a medium-size frying pan with the cooking spray; then heat the pan and add the onion and sauté until it is transparent. Add green pepper and mushrooms and sauté until they are tender. Pour in the tomato sauce and simmer over medium heat for 10 minutes. Spray a 6-inch-square baking pan with cooking spray. Line the bottom with a layer of lasagna noodles. Spread layer of all the vegetables evenly over the lasagna, and top with the tomato sauce. Then evenly distribute a layer of ricotta cheese over the vegetable–sauce mixture. Make a top layer with the remaining lasagna noodles and spread the mozzarella cheese over the noodles. Bake for 45 minutes.

Cinnamon Mousse

MAKES 4 SERVINGS (40 CALORIES EACH)

1 *cup prepared Dream Whip*
2 *egg whites*
½ *teaspoon cream of tartar*
2 *teaspoons low-calorie vanilla pudding powder*
1 *teaspoon ground cinnamon*
2 *tablespoons water*

Beat the egg whites and cream of tartar in a small mixing bowl with an electric mixer at high speed until stiff peaks form. Add pudding powder, cinnamon, and water to the prepared Dream Whip and mix well; then fold in the beaten egg whites. Spoon into serving dishes and chill for 1 hour before serving.

Liver Pâté

MAKES 4 SERVINGS (40 CALORIES EACH)

¼ *pound chicken liver*
1 *teaspoon chopped garlic*
1 *teaspoon chopped onion*
1 *teaspoon chopped celery*
1 *teaspoon chopped fresh parsley leaves*
Dash of dried thyme
Dash of black pepper
¼ *teaspoon dry mustard*
1 *tablespoon low-sodium chicken broth*
Lettuce leaves and tomato slices

Braise the chicken livers, onion, and celery in the broth in a nonstick skillet for 8 to 12 minutes. Drain off the juice and purée with the remaining ingredients (except the lettuce and tomato slices), in blender. Transfer to a bowl, cover, and refrigerate. Serve on lettuce leaves and garnish with a tomato slice.

Shredded Carrot Salad

MAKES 1 SERVING (40 CALORIES)

½ *cup shredded carrot*
1 *lettuce leaf*
2 *tablespoons Yogurt-Pineapple Dressing (recipe below)*

Arrange the carrots on the lettuce leaf and drizzle with the salad dressing before serving.

Yogurt-Pineapple Dressing

MAKES 2 TBSP. (APPROXIMATELY 30 CALORIES EACH)
½ cup plain lowfat yogurt
¼ cup unsweetened pineapple juice

Blend the ingredients well, cover, and chill before serving.

Stuffed Chicken Suprême

MAKES 4 SERVINGS (200 CALORIES EACH)
1 cup Fiber Dressing (see recipe page 199)
4 4-ounce chicken breasts, skinned and boned
Vegetable cooking spray (Pam)
1 cup Chicken Sauce (recipe below)
Chopped fresh parsley leaves

Put an equal amount of dressing on each chicken breast. Roll up the breasts to enclose the dressing and secure with toothpicks. Place the rolled breasts in a small baking pan lightly sprayed with the cooking spray. Bake for 30 minutes. Remove the breasts from the oven and transfer to a serving plate. Spoon 4 tablespoons (¼ cup) of the Chicken Sauce over each portion and garnish with the parsley.

Chicken Sauce

MAKES APPROXIMATELY 1 CUP (10 CALORIES PER OUNCE)
1 cup low-sodium chicken broth
4 teaspoons arrowroot
2 tablespoons skim milk

Bring the stock to a boil in a small saucepan. Mix the arrowroot with the milk and add slowly to stock while whipping vigorously with wire whisk. Cook just until the sauce has thickened.

Apricot Snow

MAKES 8 SERVINGS (40 CALORIES EACH)
¾ cup dried apricots
1½ cups boiling water
1 envelope unflavored gelatin
¼ cup cold water
⅓ cup apple juice concentrate
½ cup unsweetened orange or pineapple juice
3 egg whites

Put the apricots in a saucepan and cover with the boiling water. Allow to stand for 1 hour. After the apricots have softened, simmer them over medium heat for 20 to 30 minutes. Cool and then purée the mixture in a food processor or blender. Return the purée to the saucepan. Soften the gelatin in the cold water and add it to the purée. Then stir in the concentrate and juice and heat the mixture for 2 to 3 minutes. Beat the egg whites with an electric mixer until stiff and fold into the apricot mixture. Spoon into ½-cup serving dishes and chill until firm.

DAY VII: MENUS

Breakfast	Calories
½ cup fresh strawberries	50
Cheese Blintz with Pineapple	200
Decaffeinated coffee or rose hips tea	0
	250

Lunch	Calories
Asparagus Spears	40
Spinach and Mushroom Salad	20
Turkey Divan served with rice	175
Fruit Torte	40
Decaffeinated coffee or rose hips tea	0
	275

Dinner	Calories
Tomato Soup	40
Garden Salad	20
Shrimp Rockefeller	230
½ cup yellow squash	20
Chocolate–Mocha Mousse	40
Decaffeinated or rose hips tea	0
	350

DAY VII: RECIPES

**Cheese Blintz
with Pineapple**

MAKES 1 SERVING (200 CALORIES)

2 prepared crêpes (see recipe page 187), at room temperature
3 ounces lowfat cottage cheese
2 tablespoons canned crushed unsweetened pineapple, warmed

Spread each crêpe with 1½ ounces of lowfat cottage cheese, top with 1 tablespoon of the pineapple and roll up the crêpe. If necessary, use low-calorie sweetener to taste.

**Chilled
Asparagus
Spears**

MAKES 1 SERVING (40 CALORIES)

5 asparagus spears
Lettuce or other greens
Lemon wedge

Steam and chill the asparagus. Arrange them on the greens and garnish with the lemon wedge.

**Spinach and
Mushroom Salad**

MAKES 2 SERVINGS (20 CALORIES EACH)

1½ cups fresh spinach leaves with stems removed, washed
4 large fresh mushrooms
2 tablespoons low-calorie salad dressing or fresh lemon juice

Pull the spinach leaves into bite-size pieces and divide between 2 bowls. Slice the mushrooms and lay the slices over the spinach. Chill well. Drizzle with the salad dressing or lemon juice before serving.

Turkey Divan

MAKES 4 SERVINGS (175 CALORIES EACH)

2 cups chopped fresh broccoli
4 4-ounce portions sliced raw, skinned, and boned turkey breast
Vegetable cooking spray (Pam)
1 cup Chicken Sauce (see recipe, page 205)
Chopped fresh parsley leaves
2 cups hot cooked rice

Preheat the oven to 325 degrees. Put equal amounts of the broccoli evenly over the turkey breast slices. Roll up the slices and secure them with toothpicks. Place the rolls in a small baking pan which has been lightly sprayed with cooking spray. Bake for 30 minutes. Remove the breasts from the oven and transfer to a serving plate. Spoon 4 tablespoons (¼ cup) of the Chicken Sauce over each portion and garnish with the parsley. Serve each roll with ½ cup rice.

Fruit Torte	MAKES 8 SERVINGS (40 CALORIES EACH) 1 *8-ounce can low-calorie fruit cocktail* 1 *envelope lemon-flavored low-calorie gelatin powder* 1 *package ladyfingers* 1 *cup prepared Dream Whip*

Drain the fruit cocktail and measure the syrup; then add enough water to make 1 cup of liquid. Bring the liquid to a boil and stir in the lemon gelatin powder until it has dissolved. Stir in 1 cup of ice and water and continue stirring until the ice melts. Chill the gelatin until it is very thick. Line an 8- by 4-inch pan with split ladyfingers. Beat the gelatin with an electric mixer until it has doubled in volume; then blend in the Dream Whip and drained fruit cocktail. Spoon over the ladyfingers in the pan, cover, and chill thoroughly before serving.

Tomato Soup	MAKES 2 SERVINGS (40 CALORIES EACH) 1 *cup low-sodium tomato juice* ½ *cup low-sodium chicken broth* *Mrs. Dash seasoning mix* *Black pepper*

Combine the juice and broth and bring to a boil. Simmer for 20 minutes and add seasoning to taste.

Garden Salad	See recipe page 187.

| Shrimp Rockefeller | MAKES 4 SERVINGS (210 CALORIES EACH) |

Shrimp Rockefeller

MAKES 4 SERVINGS (210 CALORIES EACH)

2 cups chopped steamed spinach
Vegetable cooking spray (Pam)
1/4 cup diced onion
1/2 teaspoon Pernod
12 ounces peeled and deveined shrimp
1/2 cup Mornay Sauce (recipe on page 213)

Put the spinach in a strainer to drain off the excess water. Lightly spray a small frying pan with the cooking spray and sauté the onion until it is transparent. Add the spinach and Pernod to the onion and mix well. Simmer for 5 minutes. Steam the shrimp for 3 minutes. To serve, put 1/2 cup of the spinach mixture on each dinner plate. Lay 3 ounces of shrimp on top and spoon 2 tablespoons of Mornay Sauce over the shrimp.

Chocolate Mocha Mousse

MAKES 4 SERVINGS (40 CALORIES EACH)

2 egg whites
1/2 teaspoon cream of tartar
2 teaspoons diet chocolate pudding powder
2 tablespoons water
1 teaspoon decaffeinated instant coffee powder
1 cup prepared Dream Whip

Put the egg whites and cream of tartar in small mixing bowl and beat with an electric mixer until stiff peaks form. Stir the pudding powder, water, and coffee into the Dream Whip and mix well. Then fold in the beaten egg whites. Chill before serving.

ADDITIONAL PALM-AIRE MENU CHOICES

These may be substituted any day. Limit your choices to between 200 and 250 calories.

SUBSTITUTE BREAKFAST CHOICES

FRUITS (40 CALORIES)
Orange juice (3 1/2 ounces)
Melon in season (1 3- to 4-inch wedge)
Berries in season (1/2 cup)
1/2 grapefruit

Grapefruit juice (4 ounces)
Cranberry juice (5 ounces)
Vegetable juice (8 ounces)
½ cup mixed fresh fruits

BREADS (70 CALORIES)
1 slice wheat toast
½ bagel, cut into thin slices
1 slice multigrain toast
Bran muffin (see recipe page 194; 75 calories)

CEREALS (CALORIES AS MARKED PER 1 CUP)
Shredded Wheat (80)
Puffed Wheat (40)
Special K (70)
Product 19 (80)
Corn Flakes (80)
Bran Flakes (90)
Rice Krispies (70)
Raisin Bran (110)
Hot grain cereal (70)

DAIRY (40 CALORIES)
½ cup skim milk
3 ounces plain lowfat yogurt
2 ounces lowfat cottage cheese

EGGS (75 CALORIES)
Poached egg
Jarlsberg Egg White Omelet (see recipe page 183)
Vegetable Egg White Omelet

SUBSTITUTE LUNCH CHOICES

APPETIZERS (40)
Melon (1 3- to 4-inch wedge)
Vegetable juice (8 ounces)

SANDWICHES (ON WHOLE WHEAT BREAD OR IN PITA BREAD, 175 CALORIES)
Chicken salad (follow the recipe for tuna salad on page 191, substituting chicken for the tuna)
Turkey breast, 2½ ounces with shredded lettuce and tomato slices
Roast beef, 2 ounces with shredded lettuce and tomato

Dill Dressing	MAKES APPROXIMATELY 3 CUPS (1 TABLESPOON = 10 CALORIES)

3 cups plain lowfat yogurt
1 ½ teaspoons black pepper
1 ½ teaspoons garlic powder
Dash of Tabasco sauce
Dash of Worcestershire sauce
½ cup chopped fresh dill

Mix all ingredients together with wire whisk. |

Cucumber Dressing	MAKES APPROXIMATELY 3 CUPS (1 TABLESPOON = 13 CALORIES)

1 cucumber
3 cups plain lowfat yogurt
1 ½ teaspoons black pepper
1 ½ teaspoons garlic powder
Dash of Tabasco sauce

Grind the cucumber in a food processor. Transfer to a bowl and combine with the yogurt and spices; mix well. |

Blue Cheese–Buttermilk Dressing	MAKES APPROXIMATELY 1 ½ CUPS (1 TABLESPOON = 25 CALORIES)

8 ounces lowfat cottage cheese
¼ cup lowfat buttermilk
1 ounce ripe blue cheese
1 teaspoon Mrs. Dash seasoning mix
1 teaspoon fresh lemon juice

Blend all the ingredients in a blender until creamy smooth. This dressing is also delicious as a dip and a topping for baked potatoes. |

Tarragon Chicken Breast

MAKES 4 SERVINGS (180 CALORIES EACH)
4 4-ounce skinless chicken breasts
1 cup Chicken Sauce (see recipe page 205)
1 tablespoon ground tarragon
Vegetable cooking spray (Pam)

Preheat the oven to 325 degrees. Lightly spray a small baking pan with the cooking spray. Put the chicken breasts in the pan and bake for 30 minutes. While the chicken is baking, put the sauce and tarragon in a small saucepan and cook over low heat. Spoon 4 tablespoons (¼ cup) of the sauce on each portion of chicken before serving.

Sherried Chicken Livers

MAKES 4 SERVINGS (205 CALORIES EACH)
1 cup cooking sherry
1 cup chopped onion
½ pound chicken livers
1 cup low-sodium tomato sauce
2 cups hot cooked rice

Heat ½ cup of the sherry in a medium-size frying pan until reduced by half. Add the onion to the sherry and sauté until the onion is transparent. Remove the onion from the pan and add the remaining sherry to the warm pan. Once the sherry starts reducing, add the chicken livers and cook until they are fully browned. Drain off any excess liquid and then add the tomato sauce and onion. Simmer until the sauce is hot. Place ½ cup of rice on each dinner plate and ladle an equal amount of chicken livers over each serving.

Lobster Pernod

MAKES 4 SERVINGS (165 CALORIES EACH)
4 6-ounce lobster tails (with shell)
1 tablespoon Pernod
4 tablespoons skim milk

Preheat the oven to 350 degrees. Cut each tail in half and drape the meat over the shell. Combine the Pernod with the skim milk and moisten each tail with 1 tablespoon of the mixture. Place the tails in a small roasting pan partially filled with water. Cover the pan with aluminum foil and bake for 8 to 10 minutes.

Eggplant Parmesan

MAKES 4 SERVINGS (175 CALORIES EACH)

Vegetable cooking spray (Pam)
1 pound eggplant, sliced thin
4 ounces part-skim mozzarella cheese, grated
1 cup low-sodium tomato sauce, heated
2 cups hot cooked rice

Preheat the oven to 350 degrees. Lightly spray a small frying pan with the cooking spray and sauté the eggplant slices over medium heat until browned on both sides. Lay the cooked eggplant in a lightly sprayed baking pan and top with the grated mozzarella. Bake for 5 minutes. Remove from the oven, and spoon 4 tablespoons (¼ cup) of warm tomato sauce over each serving. Serve each portion with ½ cup of rice.

Mornay Sauce

MAKES 2 CUPS (20 CALORIES PER OUNCE)

1 cup Chablis wine
2 tablespoons arrowroot
2 teaspoons herb seasoning
1 cup skim milk
2 ounces Jarlsberg cheese, shredded

Put the wine in a saucepan and bring to a boil; then remove from the heat. Combine the arrowroot and herb seasoning with the skim milk and add to the heated wine. Add the shredded Jarlsberg slowly, whipping with a wire whisk constantly until it is fully melted.

213

Stuffed Green Peppers with Jarlsberg Cheese

MAKES 4 SERVINGS (185 CALORIES EACH)

2 large sweet green peppers
Vegetable cooking spray
½ cup chopped onion
½ cup chopped fresh mushrooms
8 ounces low-sodium tomato sauce
2 cups cooked rice
4 ounces Jarlsberg cheese, grated

Cut each pepper in half lengthwise and remove the seeds. Steam for 3 minutes. Remove and run under cold water. Lightly spray a small frying pan with the cooking spray and place over medium heat. Add the onion and sauté until transparent; then add the mushrooms. Once the mushrooms are tender, add the tomato sauce and rice to the pan and lower the heat. Simmer for 5 minutes, stirring occasionally. Fill each pepper with equal amounts of rice mixture. Sprinkle 1 ounce of Jarlsberg cheese on top of each stuffed pepper and bake for 5 minutes.

Seafood Creole à la Pomme

MAKES 4 SERVINGS (210 CALORIES EACH)

4 medium-size potatoes
Vegetable cooking spray (Pam)
½ medium-size onion, diced
½ cup chopped sweet green pepper
½ cup sliced fresh mushrooms
8 ounces low-sodium tomato sauce
¼ pound scallops
¼ pound shrimp
2 ounces Jarlsberg cheese, shredded

Bake the potatoes in a 425-degree oven for 1 hour. Remove the potatoes from the oven and let them cool. Slice an elongated strip from the top portion of each potato. Take out the "meat" of the potato without piercing the skin and discard. Set the skins aside. Sauté the onion in a lightly sprayed frying pan until it is transparent. Add the pepper and mushrooms and sauté. Stir in the tomato sauce and seafood and simmer for 10 minutes. Put equal amounts of the shrimp, scallops, and creole sauce in each potato shell. Top each shell with 1 tablespoon of cheese and bake in the oven for 5 minutes.

Tomato Sauce

16 *ounces canned whole peeled low-sodium tomatoes*
16 *ounces low-sodium tomato juice*
1 *small potato*
1 *teaspoon dried basil*
1 *teaspoon dried oregano*
1 *teaspoon chopped fresh parsley leaves*
½ *teaspoon dried thyme*
½ *teaspoon dried marjoram*
4 *cracked bay leaves*
1 *garlic clove, pressed*

Combine the tomatoes, tomato juice, spices, and one potato (wrapped in gauze to absorb acidity) in a small pot. Bring the mixture to a boil; then lower the heat and simmer for 20 minutes.

Appendix: Nutritive Value of Foods

Science and Education Administration

U.S. DEPARTMENT OF AGRICULTURE

	AMOUNT	FOOD ENERGY (Calories)	PROTEIN (Grams)	FAT (Grams)	CARBO-HYDRATES (Grams)
DAIRY PRODUCTS					
Cheese, natural					
Blue	1 oz.	100	6	8	1
Cheddar (cut into pieces)	1 oz.	115	7	9	Trace
Creamed cottage cheese (4% fat)	1 cup	235	28	10	6
Lowfat cottage cheese (1% fat)	1 cup	165	28	2	6
Cream cheese	1 oz.	100	2	10	1
Mozzarella, made with whole milk	1 oz.	90	6	7	1
Mozzarella, made with part skim milk	1 oz.	80	8	5	1
Parmesan, grated	1 tbsp.	25	2	2	Trace
Ricotta, made with whole milk	1 cup	430	28	32	7
Ricotta, made with part skim milk	1 cup	340	28	19	13
Swiss	1 oz.	105	8	8	1
Cheese, American, pasteurized process	1 oz.	105	6	9	Trace
Cream, sweet					
Half-and-half (cream and milk)	1 tbsp.	20	Trace	2	1
Light, coffee, or table	1 tbsp.	30	Trace	3	1
Whipping, light (unwhipped—volume about double when whipped)	1 tbsp.	45	Trace	5	Trace
Whipping, heavy (unwhipped—volume about double when whipped)	1 tbsp.	80	Trace	6	Trace
Whipped topping (pressurized)	1 tbsp.	10	Trace	1	Trace
Cream, sour	1 cup	495	7	48	10
	1 tbsp.	25	3	Trace	1
Milk, fluid					
Whole (3.3% fat)	1 cup	150	8	8	11
Lowfat (1% fat), no milk solids added	1 cup	100	8	3	12
Nonfat (skim), no milk solids added	1 cup	85	8	Trace	Trace
Buttermilk	1 cup	100	8	2	12
Milk, canned					
Evaporated, unsweetened (whole milk)	1 cup	340	17	19	25
Evaporated, unsweetened (skim milk)	1 cup	200	19	1	29

217

	AMOUNT	FOOD ENERGY (Calories)	PROTEIN (Grams)	FAT (Grams)	CARBO-HYDRATES (Grams)
Sweetened, condensed	1 cup	980	24	27	166
Milk Beverages					
Chocolate milk (commercial), regular	1 cup	210	8	8	26
Chocolate shake, thick (container net weight 10.6 oz.)	1 cont.	355	9	8	63
Vanilla shake, thick (container net weight 11 oz.)	1 cont.	350	12	9	56
Milk Desserts, frozen					
Ice Cream, regular (about 11% fat)	1 cup	270	5	14	32
Ice Cream, soft serve (frozen custard)	1 cup	375	7	23	38
Sherbet (about 2% fat)	1 cup	270	2	4	.1
Milk Desserts, other					
Puddings, from mix (chocolate and milk), regular (cooked)	1 cup	320	9	8	.2
Yogurt, with added milk solids (lowfat milk)					
Fruit flavored (container net weight 6 oz.)	1 cont.	230	10	3	.1
Plain (container net weight 6 oz.)	1 cont.	145	12	4	.1
Eggs, large (24 oz. per doz.)					
Fried in butter	1 egg	85	5	6	.6
Hard-cooked (shell removed)	1 egg	80	6	6	.6
Poached	1 egg	80	6	6	.6
Scrambled in butter (milk added)—also omelet	1 egg	95	6	7	.6
FATS, OILS, RELATED PRODUCTS					
Butter (1 tbsp. = about ⅛ stick)	1 tbsp.	100	Trace	12	.3
Fats, cooking (vegetable shortenings)	1 tbsp.	110	0	13	0
Margarine, regular (1 brick or 4 sticks per lb.), about ⅛ stick	1 tbsp.	100	Trace	12	Trace
Oils, salad or cooking					
Corn Oil	1 tbsp.	120	0	14	7.8
Olive Oil	1 tbsp.	120	0	14	1.1
Peanut Oil	1 tbsp.	120	0	14	4.2
Safflower Oil	1 tbsp.	120	0	14	0.0

	AMOUNT	FOOD ENERGY (Calories)	PROTEIN (Grams)	FAT (Grams)	CARBO-HYDRATES (Grams)
Salad Dressings (commercial)					
Blue cheese, regular	1 tbsp.	75	1	8	1.6
Blue cheese, low calorie (5 cal. per tsp.)	1 tbsp.	10	Trace	1	.5
French, regular	1 tbsp.	65	Trace	6	1.1
French, low calorie (5 cal. per tsp.)	1 tbsp.	15	Trace	1	.1
Italian, regular	1 tbsp.	85	Trace	9	1.6
Italian, low calorie (2 cal. per tsp.)	1 tbsp.	10	Trace	1	.1
Mayonnaise	1 tbsp.	100	Trace	11	2.0
FISH AND SHELLFISH					
Bluefish, baked with butter or margarine	3 oz.	135	22	4	0
Clams, raw, meat only	3 oz.	65	11	1	2
Clams, canned, solids and liquid	3 oz.	45	7	1	2
Crab meat, canned, not pressed down, (white or king)	1 cup	135	24	3	1
Fish sticks, breaded, cooked, frozen (stick, 4 × 1 × ½″)	1 stick (or 1 oz.)	50	5	3	2
Haddock, breaded, fried	3 oz.	140	17	5	5
Ocean perch, breaded, fried	1 fillet	195	16	11	6
Oysters, raw, meat only (13 to 19 medium selects)	1 cup	160	20	4	8
Salmon, pink, canned, solids and liquid	3 oz.	120	17	5	0
Sardines, Atlantic, canned in oil, drained solids	3 oz.	175	20	9	0
Scallops, frozen, breaded, fried, reheated	6 scallops	175	16	8	9
Shad, baked with butter or margarine	3 oz.	170	20	10	0
Shrimp, canned meat	3 oz.	100	21	1	1
Shrimp, french fried	3 oz.	190	17	9	9
Tuna, canned, in oil, drained solids	3 oz.	170	24	7	0
Tuna salad	1 cup	350	30	22	7
MEAT AND MEAT PRODUCTS					
Bacon (20 slices per lb., raw) broiled or fried, crisp	2 slices	85	4	8	Trace

	AMOUNT	FOOD ENERGY (Calories)	PROTEIN (Grams)	FAT (Grams)	CARBO-HYDRATES (Grams)
Beef, cooked					
Cuts braised, simmered, or pot roasted					
Lean and fat (piece 2½ × 2½ × ¾″)	3 oz.	240	23	16	0
Lean only	2.5 oz.	140	22	5	0
Ground beef, broiled					
Lean with 10% fat (3 × ⅝″ patty)	3 oz.	185	23	10	0
Lean with 21% fat (3 × ⅝″ patty)	2.9 oz.	235	20	17	0
Roast beef, oven cooked, no liquid added					
Relatively fat (such as rib), lean and fat, (2 pcs. 4⅛ × 2¼ × ¼″)	3 oz.	375	17	33	0
Lean only	1.8 oz.	125	14	7	0
Relatively lean (such as heel of round), lean and fat (2 pcs. 4⅛ × 2¼ × ¼″)	3 oz.	165	25	7	0
Lean only	2.8 oz.	125	24	3	0
Steak					
Relatively fat sirloin, broiled	3 oz.	330	20	27	0
Relatively lean round, braised	3 oz.	220	24	13	0
Beef, canned					
Corned beef	3 oz.	185	22	10	0
Corned beef hash	1 cup	400	19	25	24
Beef and vegetable stew	1 cup	220	16	11	15
Beef potpie (home recipe), baked (⅓ of 9″ diam. pie)	1 piece	515	21	30	39
Chili con carne with beans, canned	1 cup	340	19	16	31
Chop suey with beef and pork (home recipe)	1 cup	300	26	17	13
Lamb, cooked					
Chop, rib (cut 3 per lb. with bone), broiled	3.1 oz.	360	18	32	0
Leg, roasted	3 oz.	235	22	16	0
Liver, beef, fried (slice 6½ × 2⅜ × ⅜″)	3 oz.	195	22	9	5
Luncheon meat					
Bologna, slice (8 per 8-oz. pkg.)	1 slice	85	3	8	Trace
Frankfurter (8 per 1-lb. pkg.), cooked (reheated)	1 frankfurter	170	7	15	1

	AMOUNT	FOOD ENERGY (Calories)	PROTEIN (Grams)	FAT (Grams)	CARBO-HYDRATES (Grams)
Ham, boiled, slice (8 per 8-oz. pkg.)	1 oz.	65	5	5	0
Ham, canned, spiced or unspiced	1 slice	175	9	15	1
Salami, cooked type, slice, (8 per 8-oz. pkg.)	1 slice	90	5	7	Trace
Pork, cured, cooked					
Ham, light cure, lean and fat, roasted (2 pieces, $4\frac{1}{8} \times 2\frac{1}{4} \times \frac{1}{4}''$)	3 oz.	245	18	19	0
Pork, fresh, cooked					
Chop, loin (cut 3 per lb. with bone), broiled	2.7 oz.	305	19	25	0
Roast, oven cooked, no liquid added	3 oz.	310	21	24	0
Veal, medium fat, cooked, bone removed					
Cutlet, ($4\frac{1}{8} \times 2\frac{1}{4} \times \frac{1}{2}''$), braised or broiled	3 oz.	185	23	9	0
Rib (2 pcs., $4\frac{1}{8} \times 2\frac{1}{4} \times \frac{1}{4}''$)	3 oz.	230	23	14	0
POULTRY AND POULTRY PRODUCTS					
Chicken, cooked					
Breast, fried, bones removed, $\frac{1}{2}$ breast (3.3 oz. with bones)	2.8 oz.	160	26	5	1
Half broiler, broiled, bones removed (10.4 oz. with bones)	6.2 oz.	240	42	7	0
Turkey, roasted, flesh, without skin					
Dark meat (piece $2\frac{1}{2} \times 1\frac{5}{8} \times \frac{1}{4}''$)	4 pieces	175	26	7	0
Light meat (piece $4 \times 2 \times \frac{1}{4}''$)	2 pieces	150	28	3	0
FRUITS AND FRUIT PRODUCTS					
Apples, fresh, unpeeled, without cores					
$2\frac{3}{4}''$ diam. (about 3 per lb. with cores)	1 apple	80	Trace	1	20
$3\frac{1}{4}''$ diam. (about 2 per lb. with cores)	1 apple	125	Trace	1	31
Apple juice, bottled or canned	1 cup	120	Trace	Trace	30
Applesauce, canned					
Sweetened	1 cup	230	1	Trace	61
Unsweetened	1 cup	100	Trace	Trace	26
Apricots					
Fresh, without pits (about 12 per lb. with pits)	3 apricots	55	1	Trace	14

	AMOUNT	FOOD ENERGY (Calories)	PROTEIN (Grams)	FAT (Grams)	CARBO-HYDRATES (Grams)
Canned in heavy syrup (halves and syrup)	1 cup	220	2	Trace	57
Dried, uncooked (28 large or 37 medium halves per cup)	1 cup	340	7	1	86
Dried, cooked, unsweetened, fruit and liquid	1 cup	215	4	1	54
Apricot nectar, canned	1 cup	145	1	Trace	37
Avocados, California, mid- and late-winter (with skin and seed, 3⅛″ diam; wt., 10 oz.)	1 avocado	370	5	37	13
Banana without peel (about 2.6 per lb. with peel)	1 banana	100	1	Trace	26
Blueberries, fresh	1 cup	90	1	1	22
Cherries					
Sour (tart), red, pitted, canned, water pack	1 cup	105	2	Trace	26
Sweet, fresh, without pits and stems	10 cherries	45	1	Trace	12
Cranberry juice cocktail, bottled, sweetened	1 cup	165	Trace	Trace	42
Cranberry sauce, sweetened, canned, strained	1 cup	405	Trace	1	104
Dates, whole, without pits	10 dates	220	2	Trace	58
Fruit cocktail, canned, in heavy syrup	1 cup	195	1	Trace	50
Grapefruit, fresh, medium, 3¾″ diam.	½ with peel	50	1	Trace	13
Grapefruit juice, canned, white, unsweetened	1 cup	100	1	Trace	24
Grapes, European type (adherent skin), fresh					
Thompson Seedless	10 grapes	35	Trace	Trace	9
Tokay and Emperor, seeded types	10 grapes	40	Trace	Trace	10
Grapejuice, canned or bottled	1 cup	165	1	Trace	42
Melons					
Cantaloupe, orange-fleshed (with rind and seed cavity, 5″ diam., 2⅓ lb.)	½ melon	80	2	Trace	20

	AMOUNT	FOOD ENERGY (Calories)	PROTEIN (Grams)	FAT (Grams)	CARBO-HYDRATES (Grams)
Honeydew (with rind and seed cavity, 6½″ diam., 5¼ lb.	¹/₁₀ melon	50	1	Trace	11
Oranges, whole, 2⅝″ diam., without peel and seeds (about 2½ per lb. with peel and seeds)	1 orange	65	1	Trace	16
Orange juice					
Fresh, all varieties	1 cup	110	2	Trace	26
Frozen concentrate, diluted with 3 parts water by volume	1 cup	120	2	Trace	29
Peaches					
Canned, yellow fleshed, solids and liquid (halves or slices)					
Canned, syrup pack	1 cup	200	1	Trace	51
Canned, water pack	1 cup	75	1	Trace	20
Fresh, whole, 2½″ diam., peeled, pitted (about 4 per pound with peels and pits)	1 peach	40	1	Trace	10
Fresh, sliced	1 cup	65	1	Trace	16
Pears					
Fresh, with skin, cored					
Bartlett, 2½″ diam. (about 2½ per lb. with cores and stems)	1 pear	100	1	1	25
Bosc, 2½″ diam. (about 3 per lb. with cores and stems)	1 pear	85	1	1	22
D'Anjou, 3″ diam. (about 2 per lb. with cores and stems)	1 pear	120	1	1	31
Canned, solids and liquid, syrup pack, heavy (halves or slices)	1 cup	195	1	1	50
Pineapple					
Fresh, diced	1 cup	80	1	Trace	21
Canned, heavy syrup pack, solids and liquid					
Canned, crushed, chunks, tidbits	1 cup	190	1	Trace	49
Canned, slices and liquid, large	1 slice	80	Trace	Trace	20
Pineapple juice, unsweetened, canned	1 cup	140	1	Trace	34
Plums					
Fresh, without pits	1 plum	30	Trace	Trace	8

223

	AMOUNT	FOOD ENERGY (Calories)	PROTEIN (Grams)	FAT (Grams)	CARBO-HYDRATES (Grams)
Canned, heavy syrup pack (Italian prunes), with pits and liquid	1 cup	215	1	Trace	56
Prunes, dried, "softenized" with pits					
Uncooked	4 extra large or 5 large	110	1	Trace	29
Cooked, unsweetened, all sizes, fruit and liquids	1 cup	255	2	1	67
Prune juice, canned or bottled	1 cup	195	1	Trace	49
Raisins, seedless					
Cup, not pressed down	1 cup	420	4	Trace	112
Packet, ½ oz. (1½ tbsp.)	1 packet	40	Trace	Trace	11
Raspberries, red					
Fresh, capped, whole	1 cup	70	1	1	17
Frozen, sweetened, 10-oz. container	1 container	280	2	1	70
Rhubarb, cooked, added sugar					
From fresh	1 cup	380	1	Trace	97
From frozen	1 cup	385	1	1	98
Strawberries					
Fresh, whole berries, capped	1 cup	55	1	1	13
Frozen, sweetened, sliced, 10-oz. container	1 container	310	1	1	79
Tangerine, fresh, 2⅜" diam. size 176, without peel (about 4 per lb. with peels and seeds)	1 tangerine	40	1	Trace	10
Watermelon, fresh, 4 × 8" wedge with rind and seeds (1/16 of 32⅔-lb. melon, 10 × 16")	1 wedge	110	2	1	27
GRAIN PRODUCTS					
Bagel, 3" diam.	1 bagel	165	6	1	30
Barley, pearled, light, uncooked	1 cup	700	16	2	158
Biscuits, baking powder, 2" diam. (enriched flour, vegetable shortening)					
From home recipe	1 biscuit	105	2	5	13
From mix	1 biscuit	90	2	3	15

	AMOUNT	FOOD ENERGY (Calories)	PROTEIN (Grams)	FAT (Grams)	CARBO-HYDRATES (Grams)
Bread crumbs (enriched), dry, grated	1 cup	390	13	5	73

Breads

	AMOUNT	FOOD ENERGY (Calories)	PROTEIN (Grams)	FAT (Grams)	CARBO-HYDRATES (Grams)
Cracked-wheat bread (¾ enriched wheat flour, ¼ cracked wheat), 18 slices per loaf	1 slice	65	2	1	13
French, enriched, slice: 5 × 2½ × 1″	1 slice	100	3	1	19
Italian, enriched, slice: 4½ × 3¼ × ¾″	1 slice	85	3	Trace	17
Raisin bread, enriched (18 slices per loaf)	1 slice	65	2	1	13
Rye bread, American light (⅔ enriched wheat flour, ⅓ rye flour), slice: 4¾ × 3¾ × ⁷⁄₁₆″	1 slice	60	2	Trace	13
Pumpernickel (⅔ rye flour, ⅓ enriched wheat flour), slice: 5 × 4 × ⅜″	1 slice	80	3	Trace	17
White bread, enriched, soft crumb type (18 slices per loaf)	1 slice	70	2	Trace	13
White bread, enriched, firm crumb type (20 slices per loaf)	1 slice	65	2	1	12
Whole wheat bread, soft crumb type (16 slices per loaf)	1 slice	65	2	1	14
Whole wheat bread, firm crumb type (18 slices per loaf)	1 slice	60	3	1	12

Breakfast cereals, hot type

	AMOUNT	FOOD ENERGY (Calories)	PROTEIN (Grams)	FAT (Grams)	CARBO-HYDRATES (Grams)
Corn (hominy) grits, degermed	1 cup	125	3	Trace	27
Farina, quick-cooking, enriched	1 cup	105	3	Trace	22
Oatmeal or rolled oats	1 cup	130	5	2	23
Wheat, rolled	1 cup	180	5	1	41
Wheat, whole-meal	1 cup	110	4	2	23

Breakfast cereals, ready-to-eat

	AMOUNT	FOOD ENERGY (Calories)	PROTEIN (Grams)	FAT (Grams)	CARBO-HYDRATES (Grams)
Bran flakes (40% bran) added sugar, salt, iron, vitamins	1 cup	105	4	1	28
Bran flakes with raisins, added sugar, salt, iron, vitamins	1 cup	145	4	1	40
Corn flakes, plain, added sugar, salt, iron, vitamins	1 cup	95	2	Trace	21
Corn flakes, sugar-coated, added salt, iron, vitamins	1 cup	155	2	Trace	37

	AMOUNT	FOOD ENERGY (Calories)	PROTEIN (Grams)	FAT (Grams)	CARBO-HYDRATES (Grams)
Corn, oat flour, puffed, added sugar, salt, iron, vitamins	1 cup	80	2	1	16
Corn, shredded, added sugar, salt, iron, thiamin, niacin	1 cup	95	2	Trace	22
Oats, puffed, added sugar, salt, minerals, vitamins	1 cup	100	3	1	19
Rice, puffed, plain, added iron, thiamin, niacin	1 cup	60	1	Trace	13
Rice, puffed, presweetened, added salt, iron, vitamins	1 cup	115	1	0	26
Wheat flakes, added sugar, salt, iron, vitamins	1 cup	105	3	Trace	24
Wheat, puffed, plain, added iron, thiamin, niacin	1 cup	55	2	Trace	12
Wheat, puffed, presweetened, added salt, iron, vitamins	1 cup	140	3	Trace	33
Wheat, shredded, plain	1 biscuit	90	2	1	20
(spoon-sized biscuits)	½ cup	90	2	1	20
Wheat germ, without salt and sugar, toasted	1 tbsp.	25	2	1	3

Cakes made from cake mixes with enriched flour

	AMOUNT	FOOD ENERGY (Calories)	PROTEIN (Grams)	FAT (Grams)	CARBO-HYDRATES (Grams)
Angel food (¹/₁₂ of cake)	1 piece	135	3	Trace	32
Coffeecake (¹/₆ of cake)	1 piece	230	5	7	38
Cupcakes, made with egg, milk, 2½″ diam., without icing	1 cupcake	90	1	3	14
Cupcakes, made with egg, milk, 2½″ diam., with chocolate icing	1 cupcake	130	2	5	21
Devil's food with chocolate icing (¹/₁₆ of cake)	1 piece	235	2	8	40
Devil's food cupcake, with chocolate icing, 2½″ diam.	1 cupcake	120	2	4	20
Gingerbread (¹/₉ of cake)	1 piece	175	2	4	32
White, 2 layer with chocolate icing (¹/₁₆ of cake)	1 piece	250	3	8	45
Yellow, 2 layer with chocolate icing (¹/₁₆ of cake)	1 piece	235	3	8	40

	AMOUNT	FOOD ENERGY (Calories)	PROTEIN (Grams)	FAT (Grams)	CARBO-HYDRATES (Grams)
Spice, $^1\!/_{17}$ of loaf	1 slice	160	2	10	16
Spongecake ($^1\!/_{12}$ of cake)	1 piece	195	5	4	36

Cookies made with enriched flour

	AMOUNT	FOOD ENERGY	PROTEIN	FAT	CARBO-HYDRATES
Brownies, ($1^3\!/_4'' \times 1^3\!/_4'' \times ^7\!/_8''$) with nuts from home recipe	1 brownie	95	1	6	10
Brownies, ($1^3\!/_4'' \times 1^3\!/_4'' \times ^7\!/_8''$) with nuts from commercial recipe	1 brownie	85	1	4	13
Chocolate chip, commercial, $2^1\!/_4''$ diam., $^3\!/_8''$ thick	4 cookies	200	2	9	29
Chocolate chip, from home recipe, $2^1\!/_3''$ diam.	4 cookies	205	2	12	24
Fig bars, square ($1^5\!/_8 \times 1^5\!/_8 \times ^3\!/_8''$) or rectangular ($1^1\!/_2 \times 1^3\!/_4 \times ^1\!/_2''$)	4 cookies	200	2	3	42
Gingersnaps, $2''$ diam., $^1\!/_4''$ thick	4 cookies	90	2	2	22
Macaroons, $2^3\!/_4''$ diam., $^1\!/_4''$ thick	2 cookies	180	2	9	25
Oatmeal, with raisins, $2^5\!/_8''$ diam., $^1\!/_4''$ thick	4 cookies	235	3	8	38
Sandwich type (chocolate or vanilla) $1^3\!/_4''$ diam., $^3\!/_8''$ thick	4 cookies	200	2	9	28
Vanilla wafers, $1^3\!/_4''$ diam., $^1\!/_4''$ thick	10 cookies	185	2	6	30

Crackers

	AMOUNT	FOOD ENERGY	PROTEIN	FAT	CARBO-HYDRATES
Graham, plain, $2^1\!/_2''$ square	2 crackers	55	1	1	10
Rye wafers, whole-grain, $1^7\!/_8 \times 3^1\!/_2''$	2 wafers	45	2	Trace	10
Saltines, made with enriched flour (4 crackers per packet)	1 packet	50	1	1	8

Danish pastry (enriched flour)

	AMOUNT	FOOD ENERGY	PROTEIN	FAT	CARBO-HYDRATES
Plain without fruit or nuts, round piece about $4^1\!/_4''$ diam. $\times 1''$	1 pastry	275	5	15	30
Ounce	1 ounce	120	2	7	13

Doughnuts, made with enriched flour

	AMOUNT	FOOD ENERGY	PROTEIN	FAT	CARBO-HYDRATES
Cake type, plain, $2^1\!/_2''$ diam., $1''$ high	1 doughnut	100	1	5	13
Yeast-leavened, glazed, $3^3\!/_4''$ diam., $1^1\!/_4''$ high	1 doughnut	205	3	11	22

Macaroni, enriched, cooked, cut lengths, elbows, shells

	AMOUNT	FOOD ENERGY	PROTEIN	FAT	CARBO-HYDRATES
Firm stage (hot)	1 cup	190	7	1	39
Tender stage, cold macaroni	1 cup	115	4	Trace	24

	AMOUNT	FOOD ENERGY (Calories)	PROTEIN (Grams)	FAT (Grams)	CARBO-HYDRATES (Grams)
Tender stage, hot macaroni	1 cup	155	5	1	32
Muffins made with enriched flour, from home recipe					
Blueberry, 2⅜″ diam., 1½″ high	1 muffin	110	3	4	17
Bran	1 muffin	105	3	4	17
Corn (enriched, degermed cornmeal and flour), 2⅜″ diam., 1½″ high	1 muffin	125	3	4	19
Noodles (egg noodles), enriched, cooked	1 cup	200	7	2	37
Noodles, chow mein, canned	1 cup	220	6	11	26
Pancakes (4″ diam)					
Buckwheat, made from mix (with buckwheat and enriched flours), egg and milk added	1 cake	55	2	2	6
Plain, made from home recipe	1 cake	60	2	2	9
Pies, piecrust made with enriched flour, vegetable shortening (9″ diam.)					
Apple (⅟₇ of pie)	1 piece	345	3	15	51
Banana cream (⅟₇ of pie)	1 piece	285	6	12	40
Blueberry (⅟₇ of pie)	1 piece	325	2	15	47
Cherry (⅟₇ of pie)	1 piece	350	4	15	52
Custard (⅟₇ of pie)	1 piece	285	8	14	30
Lemon meringue (⅟₇ of pie)	1 piece	305	4	12	45
Peach (⅟₇ of pie)	1 piece	345	3	14	52
Pecan (⅟₇ of pie)	1 piece	495	6	27	67
Pumpkin (⅟₇ of pie)	1 piece	275	5	15	32
Pizza (cheese) baked, 4¾″ wedge or ⅛ of 12″ diam. pie	1 piece	145	6	4	22
Popcorn, popped					
Plain, large kernel	1 cup	25	1	Trace	5
With oil (coconut) and salt added, large kernel	1 cup	40	1	2	5
Pretzels, made with enriched flour					
Dutch, twisted, 2¾ × 2⅝″	1 pretzel	60	2	1	12
Thin, twisted, 3¼ × 2¼ × ¼″	10 pretzels	235	6	3	46
Stick, 2¼″ long	10 pretzels	10	Trace	Trace	2

	AMOUNT	FOOD ENERGY (Calories)	PROTEIN (Grams)	FAT (Grams)	CARBO-HYDRATES (Grams)
Rice, white, enriched					
Instant, ready-to-serve, hot	1 cup	180	4	Trace	40
Long-grain, cooked, served hot	1 cup	225	4	Trace	50
Rolls, enriched, commercial					
Brown-and-serve (12 per 12-oz. pkg.), browned	1 roll	85	2	2	14
Cloverleaf or pan, 2½" diam., 2" high	1 roll	85	2	2	15
Frankfurter and hamburger (8 per 11½ oz. pkg.)	1 roll	120	3	2	21
Hard, 3¾" diam., 2" high	1 roll	155	5	2	30
Hoagie or submarine, 11½ × 3 × 2½"	1 roll	390	12	4	75
Spaghetti, enriched, cooked					
Firm stage *al dente*, served hot	1 cup	190	7	1	39
Tender stage, served hot	1 cup	155	5	1	32
Spaghetti (enriched) in tomato sauce with cheese					
From home recipe	1 cup	260	9	9	37
Canned	1 cup	190	6	2	39
Spaghetti (enriched) with meat balls and tomato sauce					
From home recipe	1 cup	330	19	12	39
Canned	1 cup	260	12	10	29
Toaster pastries	1 pastry	200	3	6	36
Waffles, made with enriched flour, 7" diam.					
From home recipe	1 waffle	210	7	7	28
From mix, egg and milk added	1 waffle	205	7	8	27
LEGUMES (DRY), NUTS, SEEDS, RELATED PRODUCTS					
Almonds, shelled, slivered, not pressed down (about 115 almonds)	1 cup	690	21	62	22
Beans, red kidney	1 cup	230	15	1	42
Blackeye peas, dry, cooked (with residual cooking liquid)	1 cup	190	13	1	35
Cashew nuts, roasted in oil	1 cup	785	24	63	41

	AMOUNT	FOOD ENERGY (Calories)	PROTEIN (Grams)	FAT (Grams)	CARBO-HYDRATES (Grams)
Coconut meat, fresh, shredded or grated, not pressed down	1 cup	275	3	28	8
Lentils, whole, cooked	1 cup	210	16	Trace	39
Peanuts, roasted in oil, salted (whole, halves, chopped)	1 cup	840	37	72	27
Peanut butter	1 tbsp.	95	4	8	3
Peas, split, dry, cooked	1 cup	230	16	1	42
Pecans, chopped or pieces (about 120 large halves)	1 cup	810	11	84	17
Sunflower seeds, dry, hulled	1 cup	810	35	69	29
Walnuts, black, chopped or broken kernels	1 cup	785	26	74	19

SUGARS AND SWEETS

Cake icings

	AMOUNT	FOOD ENERGY (Calories)	PROTEIN (Grams)	FAT (Grams)	CARBO-HYDRATES (Grams)
Boiled, white, plain	1 cup	295	1	0	75
Uncooked, chocolate, made with milk and butter	1 cup	1035	9	38	185
Creamy fudge from mix and water	1 cup	830	7	16	183
White	1 cup	1200	2	21	260

Candy

	AMOUNT	FOOD ENERGY (Calories)	PROTEIN (Grams)	FAT (Grams)	CARBO-HYDRATES (Grams)
Caramels, plain or chocolate	1 oz.	115	1	3	22
Chocolate, milk, plain	1 oz.	145	2	9	16
Chocolate, semisweet, small pieces (60 per oz.; 1 cup per 6-oz. package)	1 pkg.	860	7	61	97
Chocolate-coated peanuts	1 oz.	160	5	12	11
Fondant, uncoated (mints, candy corn, other)	1 oz.	105	Trace	1	25
Fudge, chocolate, plain	1 oz.	115	1	3	21
Gumdrops	1 oz.	100	Trace	Trace	25
Hard	1 oz.	110	0	Trace	28
Marshmallows	1 oz.	90	1	Trace	23
Honey, strained or extracted	1 tbsp.	65	Trace	0	17
Jams and preserves	1 tbsp.	55	Trace	Trace	14
Jellies	1 tbsp.	50	Trace	Trace	13

	AMOUNT	FOOD ENERGY (Calories)	PROTEIN (Grams)	FAT (Grams)	CARBO-HYDRATES (Grams)
Syrups					
Chocolate-flavored syrup or topping, thin type	1 fl. oz or 2 tbsp.	90	1	1	24
Chocolate-flavored syrup or topping, fudge type	1 fl. oz. or 2 tbsp.	125	2	5	20
Molasses, cane					
Light (first extraction)	1 tbsp.	50	—	—	13
Blackstrap (third extraction)	1 tbsp.	125	—	—	11
Sugars					
Brown, pressed down	1 cup	820	0	0	212
White, granulated	1 cup	770	0	0	199
	1 tbsp.	45	0	0	12
	1 packet	23	0	0	6
Powdered	1 cup	385	0	0	100
VEGETABLES AND VEGETABLE PRODUCTS					
Asparagus, green, cooked, drained (spears ½" diam. at base, from raw)	4 spears	10	1	Trace	2
Beans, Lima, immature seeds, frozen, cooked, drained					
Thick seeded types (Fordhooks)	1 cup	170	10	Trace	32
Thin seeded types (baby limas)	1 cup	210	13	Trace	40
Beans, Green, cooked, drained, from raw (cuts and French style)	1 cup	30	2	Trace	7
Beets, cooked, drained, peeled, diced or sliced	1 cup	55	2	Trace	12
Broccoli, cooked, drained, from raw, stalk, medium size	1 stalk	45	6	1	8
Brussels sprouts, cooked, drained, from raw, 7 to 8 sprouts (1¼ to 1½" diam.)	1 cup	55	7	1	10
Cabbage, common varieties					
Raw					
Coarsely shredded or sliced	1 cup	15	1	Trace	4
Finely shredded or chopped	1 cup	20	1	Trace	5
Cooked, drained	1 cup	30	2	Trace	6

	AMOUNT	FOOD ENERGY (Calories)	PROTEIN (Grams)	FAT (Grams)	CARBO-HYDRATES (Grams)
Carrots					
Raw, without crowns and tips, scraped					
Whole, 7½ × 1⅛", or strips 2½ to 3" long	1 carrot or 18 strips	30	1	Trace	7
Grated	1 cup	45	1	Trace	11
Cooked (crosswise cuts), drained	1 cup	50	1	Trace	11
Cauliflower					
Raw, chopped	1 cup	31	3	Trace	6
Cooked, drained, from raw (flower buds)	1 cup	30	3	Trace	5
Cooked, drained, from frozen (flowerets)	1 cup	30	3	Trace	6
Celery, Pascal type, raw, stalk, large outer, 8 × 1½" at root end	1 stalk	5	Trace	Trace	2
Corn, sweet					
Cooked, drained, from raw ear, 5 × 1¾"	1 ear	70	2	1	16
Cooked, drained, from frozen ear, 5" long	1 ear	120	4	1	27
Cooked, drained, from frozen kernels	1 cup	130	5	1	31
Canned, cream style	1 cup	210	5	2	51
Canned, whole kernel, vacuum pack	1 cup	175	5	1	43
Cucumber slices, ⅛" thick (large, 2⅛" diam; small, 1¾" diam)	6 large or 8 small slices	5	Trace	Trace	1
Lettuce, raw					
Crisp head, as Iceberg, wedge, ¼ of head	1 wedge	20	1	Trace	4
Crisp head, as Iceberg, pieces, chopped or shredded	1 cup	5	Trace	Trace	2
Looseleaf (bunching varieties including romaine or cos), chopped or shredded pieces)	1 cup	10	1	Trace	2
Mushrooms, raw, sliced or chopped	1 cup	20	2	Trace	3
Okra pods, 3 × ⅝", cooked	10 pods	30	2	Trace	6

	AMOUNT	FOOD ENERGY (Calories)	PROTEIN (Grams)	FAT (Grams)	CARBO-HYDRATES (Grams)
Onions					
Mature, raw, chopped	1 cup	65	3	Trace	15
Mature, raw, sliced	1 cup	45	2	Trace	10
Peas, green					
Canned, whole, drained solids	1 cup	150	8	1	29
Frozen, cooked, drained	1 cup	110	8	Trace	19
Peppers, sweet (about 5 per lb., whole), stem and seeds removed					
Raw	1 pod	15	1	Trace	4
Cooked, boiled, drained	1 pod	15	1	Trace	3
Potatoes, cooked					
Baked, peeled after baking (about 2 per lb. raw)	1 potato	145	4	Trace	33
Boiled (about 3 per lb. raw), peeled after boiling	1 potato	105	3	Trace	23
Boiled (about 3 per lb. raw), peeled before boiling	1 potato	90	3	Trace	20
French-fried, strip 2 to 3½" long, prepared from raw	10 strips	135	2	7	18
French-fried, strip 2 to 3½" long, frozen, oven-heated	10 strips	110	2	4	17
Hashed brown, prepared from frozen	1 cup	345	3	18	45
Mashed, prepared from raw, milk added	1 cup	135	4	2	27
Mashed, prepared from raw, milk and butter added	1 cup	195	4	9	26
Potato chips, 1¾ × 2½" oval, cross section	10 chips	115	1	8	10
Potato salad, made with cooked salad dressing	1 cup	250	7	7	41
Radishes, raw (prepackaged) stem ends, rootlets cut off	4 radishes	5	Trace	Trace	1
Sauerkraut, canned, solids and liquid	1 cup	40	2	Trace	2
Spinach					
Raw, chopped	1 cup	15	2	Trace	2
Cooked, drained, from raw	1 cup	40	5	1	6

233

	AMOUNT	FOOD ENERGY (Calories)	PROTEIN (Grams)	FAT (Grams)	CARBO-HYDRATES (Grams)
Squash, cooked					
Summer (all varieties) diced, drained	1 cup	30	2	Trace	7
Winter (all varieties) baked, mashed	1 cup	130	4	1	32
Sweet potatoes, cooked (raw, 5 × 2",					
about 2½ per lb.)					
Baked in skin, peeled	1 potato	160	2	1	37
Boiled in skin, peeled	1 potato	170	3	1	40
Candied, 2½ × 2" piece	1 piece	175	1	3	36
Tomatoes					
Raw, 2⅗" diam. (3 per 12-oz. pkg.)	1 tomato	25	1	Trace	6
Canned, solids and liquid	1 cup	50	2	Trace	10
Tomato catsup	1 tbsp.	15	Trace	Trace	4
Tomato juice	8 oz.	35	2	Trace	8
Turnips, cooked, diced	1 cup	35	1	Trace	8
Vegetables, mixed, frozen, cooked	1 cup	115	6	1	24
MISCELLANEOUS					
Barbecue sauce	1 cup	230	46	17	20
Beverages, alcoholic					
Beer	12 fl. oz.	150	1	0	14
Gin, rum, vodka, whisky, 80-proof					
(1½ fl. oz. jigger)	1 jigger	95	—	—	Trace
Gin, rum, vodka, whisky, 90-proof	1 jigger	110	—	—	Trace
Wines, dessert (3½ fl. oz. glass)	1 glass	140	Trace	0	8
Wines, table (3½ fl. oz. glass)	1 glass	85	Trace	0	4
Beverages, carbonated, sweetened,					
nonalcoholic					
Cola-type	12 fl. oz.	145	0	0	37
Fruit-flavored sodas and Tom Collins					
mixer	12 fl. oz.	170	0	0	45
Ginger ale	12 fl. oz	115	0	0	29
Root beer	12 fl. oz.	150	0	0	39
Gelatin dessert prepared with gelatin					
dessert powder and water	1 cup	140	4	0	34
Mustard, prepared, yellow (1 tsp. per					
individual serving pouch or cup)	1 tsp.	5	Trace	Trace	Trace

	AMOUNT	FOOD ENERGY (Calories)	PROTEIN (Grams)	FAT (Grams)	CARBO-HYDRATES (Grams)
Olives, green, pickled, canned	4 medium, 3 ex. large, or 2 giant	15	Trace	2	Trace
Pickles, cucumber					
Dill, medium, whole, 3¾" long, 1¼" diam.	1 pickle	5	Trace	Trace	1
Sweet, gherkin, small, whole, about 2½" long, ¾" diam.	1 pickle	20	Trace	Trace	5
Relish, finely chopped, sweet	1 tbsp.	20	Trace	Trace	5
Popsicle, 3 fl. oz. size	1 pop	70	0	10	18
Soups, canned, condensed, prepared with equal volume of milk					
Cream of chicken	1 cup	180	7	10	15
Cream of mushroom	1 cup	215	7	14	16
Tomato	1 cup	175	7	7	23
Soups, canned, condensed, prepared with equal volume of water					
Beef broth, bouillon, consommé	1 cup	30	5	0	3
Beef noodle	1 cup	65	4	3	7
Clam chowder, Manhattan type (with tomatoes, without milk)	1 cup	80	2	3	12
Cream of chicken	1 cup	95	3	6	8
Cream of mushroom	1 cup	135	2	10	10
Minestrone	1 cup	105	5	3	14
Split pea	1 cup	145	9	3	21
Tomato	1 cup	90	2	3	16
Vegetable beef	1 cup	80	5	2	10
Vegetarian	1 cup	80	2	2	13
Soups, dehydrated bouillon cube, ½"	1 cube	5	1	Trace	Trace
Soups, dehydrated mixes, prepared with water					
Chicken noodle	1 cup	55	2	1	8
Onion	1 cup	35	1	1	6
Tomato vegetable with noodles	1 cup	65	1	1	12
White sauce, medium, with enriched flour	1 cup	405	10	31	22

Index

Eleanor Berman is the author of six books, on subjects as diverse as travel, child rearing, and women returning to work. She has written for *Working Mother*, *Harper's Bazaar*, and *Travel and Leisure*, among other periodicals. Ms. Berman is a graduate of Smith College and resides in New York City.

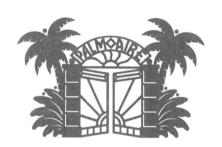

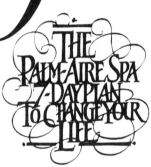

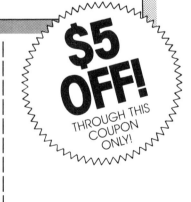